Sharon G. Mijares
Editor

Modern Psychology and Ancient Wisdom
Psychological Healing Practices from the World's Religious Traditions

Pre-publication
REVIEWS,
COMMENTARIES,
EVALUATIONS . . .

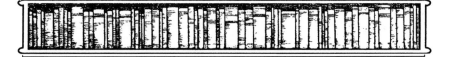

More pre-publication
REVIEWS, COMMENTARIES, EVALUATIONS . . .

"There is a great depth of information provided in this wonderful book. Each chapter illuminates well the potential of a particular spiritual discipline to enhance the practice of psychotherapy.

The book skillfully portrays the timely and enduring relevance of a vast number of wisdom traditions—Eastern, Western, and Earth based—to psychology. With vivid case examples, it enlarges the notion of psychological well-being in light of spiritual understanding and values. The detailed descriptions of each tradition trace the contours and perils of the journey of psychospiritual discovery. A must-read for therapists, spiritual and pastoral counselors, and all those who are interested in the intersection of psyche and spirit."

Daniel Deslauriers, PhD
Director, East-West Psychology Program,
California Institute of Integral Studies

"This book is a welcome resource for those who are seeking to understand more about the connection between spirituality and psychology. It will be helpful to mental health professionals, who are becoming more aware of the importance of attending to the spirituality of their clients, as well as to the growing number of professionally trained spiritual guides, who must take into account the psychology of the individuals with whom they work.

The introduction to the various religious traditions, and an articulation of the psychology inherent in each of these traditions, will enhance the healing process not only of individuals but hopefully of our diverse planet which is so much in need of healing."

Paul J. Roy, PhD
Dean, Residential Division,
Institute of Transpersonal Psychology

The Haworth Integrative Healing Press®
An Imprint of The Haworth Press, Inc.
New York • London • Oxford

Modern Psychology and Ancient Wisdom

Psychological Healing Practices from the World's Religious Traditions

THE HAWORTH INTEGRATIVE HEALING PRESS
Ethan Russo
Editor

The Last Sorcerer: Echoes of the Rainforest by Ethan Russo

Professionalism and Ethics in Complementary and Alternative Medicine by John Crellin and Fernando Ania

Cannabis and Cannabinoids: Pharmacology, Toxicology, and Therapeutic Potential by Franjo Grotenhermen and Ethan Russo

Modern Psychology and Ancient Wisdom: Psychological Healing Practices from the World's Religious Traditions edited by Sharon G. Mijares

Complementary and Alternative Medicine: Clinic Design by Robert A. Roush

Modern Psychology and Ancient Wisdom
Psychological Healing Practices from the World's Religious Traditions

Sharon G. Mijares
Editor

The Haworth Integrative Healing Press®
An Imprint of The Haworth Press, Inc.
New York • London • Oxford

Published by

The Haworth Integrative Healing Press®, an imprint of The Haworth Press, Inc., 10 Alice Street, Binghamton, NY 13904-1580.

PUBLISHER'S NOTE
Identities and circumstances of individuals discussed in this book have been changed to protect confidentiality.

Copyright acknowledgments can be found on p. xxii.

Cover design by Lora Wiggins.

Library of Congress Cataloging-in-Publication Data

Mijares, Sharon G. (Sharon Grace), 1942-
    Modern psychology and ancient wisdom : psychological healing practices from the world's religious traditions / Sharon G. Mijares.
        p. cm.
    Includes bibliographical references and index.
    ISBN 0-7890-1751-2 (alk. paper)—ISBN 0-7890-1752-0 (pbk.)
    1. Spiritual healing. I. Title.

BL65.M4 M55 2002
291.3'1—dc21

2002069085

For my children Raphael, Connie, and Christina.

They have taught me much about myself
and the power of love.

CONTENTS

ABOUT THE EDITOR

Sharon G. Mijares, PhD, is a Self-Relations Psychotherapist. She received her doctoral degree through the Union Institute (1995) and completed her postdoctoral fellowship at Mercy-Scripps Behavioral Health Care. She is a member of the Sufi Ruhaniat International, the International Association of Sufism's Psychology and Sufism Forum, and the Mentor's Training Guild of the International Network for the Dances of Universal Peace. Dr. Mijares also serves on the Advisory Board of the International Association of Sufism. She is a core adjunct faculty member of National University's Psychology Department and Chapman University's Counseling Psychology Program. She is respected for her creative approaches and successes with healing victims of sexual abuse. Dr. Mijares has been an active facilitator of women's groups and women's healing processes. She has authored several articles on spiritual emergence and the mind-body relationship, and recently contributed a chapter for Stephen Gilligan's and Dvorah Simond's edited book *Walking in Two Worlds: Theory and Practice of Self Relations.* She can be contacted at (760) 436-3518, <www. sharonmijares.com>, or <www.TheWomensCoach.com>.

CONTRIBUTORS

Eleanor Criswell, EdD, is a professor of psychology and former chair of the Psychology Department, Sonoma State University. She is the founding director of the Humanistic Psychology Institute (now Saybrook Graduate School and Research Center) and is a distinguished consulting member for Saybrook Graduate School. Dr. Criswell is editor of *Somatics: Magazine-Journal of the Mind/Body Arts and Sciences,* president of the Somatics Society, and director of the Novato Institute for Somatic Research and Training. Her books include *Biofeedback and Somatics: Toward Personal Evolution* (Freeperson Press, 1995) and *How Yoga Works: An Introduction to Somatic Yoga* (Freeperson Press, 1987). She is co-editor of *Biofeedback and Family Practice Medicine* (Perseus Publishing, 1983). A past president of the Association for Humanistic Psychology, Dr. Criswell is president of the board of directors of Division 32, the Humanistic Psychology Division of the American Psychology Association, a licensed psychologist, and a somatic educator. A practitioner of yoga psychology and meditation for thirty-five years, she has taught yoga psychology in the Psychology Department of Sonoma State University for thirty-two years. Dr. Criswell has published articles on yoga psychology in magazines and journals during that time. As editor of *Somatics: Magazine-Journal of the Mind/Body Arts and Sciences,* she has a strong interest in furthering the awareness of the possibilities of health and well-being inherent in mind-body integration. To that end she trains teachers of yoga psychology and somatic yoga.

Neil Douglas-Klotz, PhD, is an independent scholar with a doctorate in psychology and religious studies (with an emphasis in Middle Eastern languages and spirituality). He is the author of *Prayers of the Cosmos* (HarperSanFrancisco, 1990), *Desert Wisdom* (HarperSanFrancisco, 1995), and *The Hidden Gospel* (Quest, 1999), and serves on the steering committee of the Mysticism Group of the American Academy of Religion. Dr. Douglas-Klotz also serves on the advisory committee of the International Association of Sufism and is recognized as a senior guide *(murshid)* in one of the branches of the Chishtia school of Sufism, called the Sufi Islamia Ruhaniat Society. He founded the International Network for the Dances of Universal Peace and teaches internationally through this group as well as through the Abwoon Study Circle <www.abwoon.com>. His most recent psychological research was published in the anthology *Psychosis and Spirituality: Exploring the New Frontier* (Whurr Publishers, 2000), edited by Isabel Clarke. He currently lives in Edinburgh, Scotland, and codirects the Edinburgh Institute for Advanced Learning.

Reverend Dwight H. Judy, PhD, is the director of Spiritual Formation for Oakwood Spiritual Life Center in Syracuse, Indiana, where he makes his home with his wife, Ruth, and their two teenaged sons. He is also the director of Doctor of Ministry and Spiritual Formation Programs, associate professor of Spiritual Formation, for Garrett-Evangelical Theological Seminary (G-ETS) in Evanston, Illinois. He is an ordained United Methodist minister, has been licensed as a psychologist in California, and is a member of the American Association of Pastoral Counselors. He is a past president of the Association for Transpersonal Psychology. Formerly, he was an associate professor at the Institute of Transpersonal Psychology in Palo Alto, California. He is the author of *Quest for the Mystical Christ: Awakening the Heart of Faith* (OSL Publications, 2003), *Embracing God: Praying with Teresa of Avila* (Abingdon, 1996), *Christian Meditation and Inner Healing* (OSL Publications, 2000, and Crossroad, 1991), and *Healing the Male Soul: Christianity and the Mythic Journey* (Crossroad, 1992). He leads retreats in Christian prayer throughout the nation, offers training in Christian spiritual formation, and is a spiritual director for individuals. His most recent book, *Quest for the Mystical Christ,* elaborates on themes presented in his contributed chapter in this book. He has been instrumental with other faculty of G-ETS and The Upper Room in Nashville in creating a Certification in Spiritual Formation process within the United Methodist Church. For information on programs, contact Oakwood Spiritual Life Center, 702 E. Lake View Road, Syracuse, Indiana 46567.

Nick Kouris, MA, is a graduate of John F. Kennedy University in Orinda, California. Mr. Kouris completed his thesis *Masks, Paradox, and the Hero's Journey* in March 1998. He has collaborated with

Dr. Terry Tafoya since 1990, and they copresented a workshop titled "Coyote and Chaos: Native American Modalities of Healing," at the Association of Transpersonal Psychology Conference at Asilomar, California, in 1997. Through the use of mythology, symbols, and paradox, Mr. Kouris's primary focus has been to explore the relationship between Western and non-Western systems of thought and how the cognitive, emotional, and spiritual modalities of each system ultimately condition one's perception of mental health and define one's approach to healing. Mr. Kouris was a clinician for the Los Angeles Youth Network (formerly Options House), an organization that provides emergency shelter, residential treatment, and other services to at-risk teens and their families. Currently, Mr. Kouris lives in Westlake Village, California, and is an account manager for a managed mental health care provider in the San Fernando Valley of Los Angeles. He can be reached via e-mail at <nskouris@aol.com> or through Dr. Tafoya's organization, Tamanawit, UnLtd.

Sheldon Z. Kramer, PhD, is a licensed clinical psychologist in full-time private practice in La Jolla, California. He is author of numerous articles, chapters, and two books on mind-body medicine, spirituality, and psychotherapy, as well as marital and family psychotherapy. Dr. Kramer is the assistant clinical instructor of psychiatry at the University of California, San Diego, School of Medicine. He is an active international trainer of health care professionals as well as a workshop presenter to the general public. He is the author of *Transforming the Inner and Outer Family: Humanistic and Spiritual Approaches to Mind-Body Systems Therapy* (The Haworth Press, 1995) and also contributed a chapter titled "Jewish Meditation: Healing Ourselves and Our Relationships" in *Opening the Inner Gates: New Pathways to Kabbalah and Psychology* (Shambhala, 1995), edited by Edward Hoffman, PhD.

Kartikeya C. Patel, PhD, is the dean of Global Division at the Institute of Transpersonal Psychology in Palo Alto, California. He has studied, taught, published, and presented in Eastern and Western traditions and maintains a Hindu-Buddhist meditation practice. Publications include "Women, Earth, and the Goddess: A Sakta-Hindu Interpretation of Embodied Religion" (*Hypatia* 9[4]) and *Wittgenstein on Emotion and the Paradox of Negation in Nagarjuna's Philosophy.* Dr. Patel brings with him the experience of living in many different cultures and the wisdom of understanding the cultural impact on psychotherapeutic models. He can be reached via e-mail at <kpatel@itp.edu>.

Terry Tafoya, PhD, trained as a traditional Native American storyteller, is a Taos Pueblo and Warm Springs Indian. He has used American Indian ritual and ceremony in his work as a family therapist at the Interpersonal Psychotherapy Clinic, part of the University of Washington's School of Medicine in Seattle. The Washington State Department of Social and Health Services designated Dr. Tafoya the first formally recognized native healer for the state as an ethnic minority mental health specialist. Dr. Tafoya directed the Transcultural Counseling program at Evergreen State College, co-founded the National Native American AIDS Prevention Center, and created Tamanawit UnLtd., an international consulting firm. He has taught with the Kinsey Institute for the Study of Human Sexuality, Gender, and Reproduction as faculty and as an expert in Cross-Cultural Sexuality. He serves as a national consultant for the U.S. Center for Substance Abuse Prevention, and is the chief curriculum writer for the Gathering of American Indians, a national project for Native American Substance Abuse Prevention. He is on the national teaching faculty for the American Psychological Association and is on the international faculty of the Milton H. Erickson Foundation for Clinical Hypnosis and Psychotherapy. Dr. Tafoya has presented over a thousand keynotes, lectures, and workshops throughout the United States, Canada, Mexico, and Europe. He can be reached by phone at (206) 632-8124, via e-mail at <Tamanawit@aol.com>, or online at <www.tamanawit.com>.

Benjamin R. Tong, PhD, is an associate professor, clinical psychology program, California Institute of Integral Studies, San Francisco; and is faculty emeritus in Asian American Studies at San Francisco State University. He is a teacher of Tai Ch'i and Qigong (School of Taoist Internal Arts); a feng shui consultant; a psychotherapist in private practice; and the executive director, Institute for Cross-Cultural Research (ICCR), a nonprofit organization that provides education, consultation, and research on indigenous health and healing arts. He has conducted workshops and symposia on a variety of cross-cultural and East/West mind-body therapy themes in both the United States and Canada. Dr. Tong is also on the board of advisors, International

Karen Horney Society, which in recent years has translated the works of Horney into Russian and Chinese. Dr. Tong can be reached via e-mail at <lohfu@yahoo.com>.

Karen Kissel Wegela, PhD, has studied and practiced Buddhism since 1972. Currently, she is a member of Naropa University's faculty leadership team of the master's in psychology: contemplative psychotherapy program and the author of *How to Be a Help Instead of a Nuisance* (Shambhala, 1996). She also writes a regular column for the *Shambhala Sun* magazine. Dr. Wegela is a psychologist and has worked with a variety of psychotherapy clients in a number of different settings. Presently, she has a private practice and also volunteers as a consultant to the staff of Friendship House, a residential treatment program for people living with severe mental disturbance. She can be reached through Naropa University, 2130 Arapahoe Avenue, Boulder, Colorado 80302, by phone at (303) 444-0202, or online at <www. naropa.edu>.

Foreword

As the saying goes, the road narrows with time. As we grow older, we pay for our mistakes more dearly. A loss is more costly; the stakes are higher; the room for error is much less. This applies not only to individuals but to the whole of humanity. We neglect our environment at the risk of destroying it. We ignore our traditions at the risk of losing them. We deal violently with differences at the risk of mutual annihilation. Today's world is so interconnected, so technologically powerful, so intimately small that truly, as the example in chaos theory poetically suggests, the flapping wings of a butterfly in Asia can affect weather patterns over Europe.

In such times, two challenges are especially immense. The first is recognizing and cultivating traditions that make us more compassionate, more aware, and perhaps a bit more wise. With so much stress in an uncertain, rapidly changing world, we must find ways to center, to breathe, to listen deeper, and to love more clearly. Because there are many paths for doing this, none inherently superior to the others, we face a second challenge of dealing with these differences. You're a Jew, and I'm not. You wear those funny clothes, and I don't. You don't believe or practice what I "know" to be the Truth, and that disturbs me.

So these two challenges—cultivating spiritual traditions that resonate with contemporary consciousness and forging new ways of creatively dealing with how differences bump up against one another—require both a connection to the past and its ancestral knowledge and an openness to a future that allows transtraditional (you might say "world beat") consciousness. Sharon Mijares has addressed both these challenges in assembling this wonderful book on religious and psychological approaches. As I read it, I had the feeling of sitting raptly at a weaving ritual of multitudinous dimensions. Each chapter evokes a particular type of reverence, a special type of vibration, a unique feeling of wisdom and hope. When held together, they create a textured symphony of enlightened consciousness. You cannot help but feel hopeful about a future that allows all these different voices to be spoken in concert.

In the present challenging times, this book is a great gift. It shares historical roots, provides general frameworks, and offers specific and practical techniques by which we can both heal psychological woundedness and deepen spiritual awareness. I hope and trust that others will benefit from it as I have.

Stephen Gilligan
Psychologist and Author
Encinitas, California

Acknowledgments

I want to express my appreciation to the contributing authors for their willingness to trust my vision and offer their time, effort, and knowledge. Without them this work would not have been possible.

I also want to take this opportunity to particularly thank the significant teachers in my life whose influences have provided the foundation for this book. First, I'd like to thank Michael Wolk, MD, for believing in me. His authentic caring, wisdom, and support allowed me to move from psychological distress to spiritual awakening. He was the one who helped me open the first door and I will always be grateful to him. Next, I'd like to thank the Reverend Flower A. Newhouse. Through her influence I recognized the importance of balancing spiritual beliefs and practices with psychological experience and behaviors. Saadi Neil Douglas-Klotz is not only a treasured friend, but also my guide on the Sufi path. My life has been and continues to be deeply blessed by his influence. He has been with me throughout my academic, professional, and spiritual development. I'd also like to thank my psychotherapy mentor, Stephen Gilligan. The last eleven years of supervision training with Steve have significantly enriched my understanding of meaningful psychotherapy. His theory of self-relations psychotherapy has melded well with my spiritual training and enriched my work with clients. I also thank my sensei, Coryl Crane, for all that she, the dojo, and the practice of aikido have provided in my life. The regular practice of aikido has helped me maintain a needed balance in the midst of the many hours spent in front of a computer. During this entire period of my life I have also had a tremendous amount of support from the International Association of Sufism and its cofounders Dr. Nahid Angha and Dr. Ali Kianfar. They have supported the unity of psychological and spiritual development.

The North County Women's Circle has been wonderful during this entire process. I love this group of women! Their strength, wisdom, and beauty empowered my chapter on the healing effects of goddess stories for women. Cass Dalglish's friendship, editorial suggestions, and expertise in Sumerian literature were priceless resources. Even though his own life was very full, the late Pir Moineddin Jablonski (1942-2001), made time to assist me with editorial suggestions. I will always be grateful to him for his kindness, love, wisdom, and practical knowledge. I also want to acknowledge my appreciation for Nicolee Miller and Dania Brett's editorial comments. Theirs was truly a labor of love. Beatrice Ring put in many hours to help me find the religious symbols placed at the beginning of each chapter. This was not an easy task, and I am very appreciative of her friendship, diligence, and support. Patti Kizzar and Kiersten Payne's help with the index is acknowledged with heartfelt appreciation.

The Haworth Press staff has been incredible. The clear organization, prompt responses, and, most important, warm and supportive editorial, administrative, and advertising staff have contributed to a very good experience. Senior editor Peg Marr always answered any questions within less than twenty-four hours. This support helped me glide easily through the early stages of production. This has also been my experience with production editor Amy Rentner. Senior editor Dawn Krisko's quick, supportive responses were also greatly appreciated, especially her guidance throughout the indexing process. I will remember Peg, Amy, and Dawn with warmth and appreciation. Thanks to all the Haworth staff who helped bring this book to fruition.

Most of all, I want to thank and acknowledge all of my clients. Their courage, dedication, creativity, and beauty will always inspire me.

COPYRIGHT ACKNOWLEDGMENTS

Excerpt from *Tao Te Ching* by Lao Tsu, translated by Gia-Fu Feng and Jane English, copyright ©1997 by Jane English. Copyright ©1972 by Gia-Fu Feng and Jane English. Used by permission of Alfred A. Knopf, a division of Random House, Inc.

Excerpt from *Talking Zen: Written and Spoken by Alan Watts,* edited by Mark Watts, ©1994 by Weatherhill. Reprinted by permission.

Excerpt from *Final Lectures* by Karen Horney, edited by Douglas H. Ingram, MD. Copyright ©1987 by the Association for the Advancement of Psychoanalysis of the Karen Horney Psychoanalytic Institute & Center. Used by permission of W. W. Norton & Company, Inc.

Extract from *The Principal Upanishads* by Radharishnan, 1953. Reprinted by permission of HarperCollins Publishers Ltd.

Extract from *Desert Wisdom: Sacred Middle Eastern Writings from the Goddess Through the Suffis,* translations and commentary by Neil Douglas-Klotz. Copyright ©1995 by Neil Douglas-Klotz. Reprinted by permission of HarperCollins Publishers, Inc.

Introduction

We have entered a new millennium. It is one of the most tumultuous and yet promising times of human history. We are also rapidly progressing in psychological understanding and expanding our knowledge of human behaviors in many ways. There are many different theories and practices of psychotherapy today, and increasing numbers of people are entering psychotherapy to heal and to change their lives. Yet why is there so much discontent with self, and why so many broken relationships? Despite the vast scientific research into human behavior and its influence on modern psychology, many people today lack a sound sense of direction in their lives. Great numbers of people live in isolation—people whose individual lives frequently touch the depths of despair. Psychology has worked diligently to understand and treat behaviors that negatively affect individuals and those surrounding them. Its theories and findings have been implemented in individual, relational, and educational realms, yet our society keeps declining. What is lacking?

Increasing numbers of people are hungry for perspectives that offer deeper meaning in life, for ways to live that reveal the soul. This hunger is evidenced in the manifold varieties of addictive behaviors affecting humanity. Why are so many people motivated to alter their consciousness? What are they seeking? They long for something more than their mundane and circumscribed lives. Many professionals feel the spiritual element has been missing and that we will never be content until we know our inherent unity with the Divine Presence from which all life manifests. In our search for ways to help those who are suffering, we have neglected to include thousands of years of well-researched healing processes and knowledge gleaned from the world's wisdom and spiritual traditions. Psychotherapists and religious practitioners need to work together to provide an integrative approach to enhance our psychological and spiritual development. Even though psychology has contributed a great deal to understanding human behavior, it has generally operated within a limited paradigm.

The teachings of the wisdom and spiritual traditions and the great prophets are now readily available, for the first time in history, to those who seek them. Throughout this century spiritual teachers from many parts of the world have come to the United States to share their wisdom. As a result, we have been blessed with teachings from around the globe to help us through this time of challenge. It is time to apply what we have been given. This knowledge, coupled with the discoveries of psychology, will help heal individuals, families, communities, and humanity as we delve more deeply into this new millennium.

After centuries of separation and antagonism, psychology and religion are at long last entering into a meaningful dialogue. Whereas psychology is a science that addresses mental, emotional, somatic, and relational dynamics, spirituality illuminates the inherent mystery of life itself. Each approach provides a perspective that completes the other. We need to listen to this shared conversation, for it affords new understandings to heal and to advance our psychological and spiritual development.

A strengthened dialogue, even a communion, between psychology and religion is needed. When we examine the following historical contributions, statistics, resulting problems, and suggested resolutions, we will find that there is a great need for this new paradigm of psychospirituality.

The World Almanac and Book of Facts 1997 reveals that over 4.5 billion persons in a worldwide human population of 6 billion people (75 percent) adhere to some form of spiritual or religious belief (1996). That is a very significant percentage, yet the field of psychology has tended to focus primarily on problems and pathological states while ignoring obvious and plentiful healing resources from the field of spirituality. Because of this limited perspective, psychotherapists have by and large received an unfortunately restricted education. The result is that many fail to listen to the deeper needs of their clients and to affirm their clients' subtle and spiritual experiences.

During my postdoctoral training in a psychiatric hospital unit, I met a very lovely, creative, and troubled woman. She had been in and out of psychiatric care since early adulthood. As with many other persons, her childhood had been very difficult. Her father had been terrifying and oppressive. He had often misconstrued the Bible by using it to support his abusive behaviors. As a young child, violence, confusion, and fear had threatened her.

Yet a light became visible in the midst of this darkness. The Archangel Michael appeared to her to reassure her that she was not alone, that angels were watching over her. She was given directions to write the story of her life. As she grew into a young woman she remained faithful to this experience into adulthood. It provided inner strength and conviction. She soon experienced a nervous breakdown due to the buildup of anxiety and fear from her childhood experiences. When she turned to the psychiatric profession for help, she told them of St. Michael's guidance.

Now, "hearing voices" is not acceptable in Western culture. It is considered to be a sign of pathology. Despite the fact that she did not report a "voice keeping up a running commentary," she was given a diagnosis of schizophrenia. But she remained faithful to her early guidance and refused to accept it as a "delusional" state.

She could not trust her caretakers as a child and she was unable to trust the professionals who could have helped her as a young woman. Although there was considerable experiential support for her resulting paranoia, it was viewed as further evidence for the diagnosis of schizophrenia. Perhaps the result would have been different if the professionals treating her had not negated her experience. Instead of insisting that she acknowledge her "symptoms," simple listening and acceptance could have opened the door to her soul. It would have encouraged trust in the therapeutic relationship.

Her boyfriend was abusive; domestic violence was suspected. Due to her mistrust of psychotherapeutic assistance, she rejected their advice and remained with him. In the spring of 1997, the local newspapers reported her murder and her partner's suicide. A few months before her death, she asked in a group therapy session if "a mental health patient ever had any credibility in this society." Perhaps she would be alive today if the professionals had listened to and accepted her experience.

Carl Jung might have called the woman's visitation an archetypal experience. It would be a profound act of creative power for a child to evoke the warrior Archangel Michael from the depths of the collective unconscious to support her in a time of need. Was this experience a sign of psychopathology, or did it bear witness to the depth and resourcefulness of the soul?

Sacred texts such as the Bible, Torah, and Qu'ran acknowledge and affirm personal visitations from angels. Many popular books describe encounters with angels experienced by a broad range of human beings. The 1996 Gallup poll reported that approximately 72 percent of the U.S. population believe in angels, 11 percent were unsure, and 1 percent had no opinion (1997). In this poll only 16 percent denied the existence of angels. It is significant that the belief in angels has remained strong despite the emphasis on scientific proof and cognitive development.

Conversely, it is also true that many persons choose alternative therapies and seek religious experiences rather than acknowledge that they have psychological problems. Although supernatural presences and nonordinary experiences are acknowledged by a multitude of people, these experiential realms present a clinical problem when persons use them to avoid unresolved pain hidden in the recesses of the psyche. Defenses such as repression, denial, rationalization, and projection protect the fragile ego but limit the untapped inner and outer potential. Traditionally, religion has emphasized denial of the human body and its wants and needs in preference for a more saint-like or transcendent ideal. This imbalanced presentation has activated repression, denial, and other defense mechanisms in many people. We believed that if we had sufficient faith, served others, sacrificed, meditated, prayed, and performed enough spiritual practices we would ultimately avoid the pitfalls of human experience and find God. Instead, many spiritual leaders, practitioners, and devotees now find themselves continuously—and uncomfortably—being reminded of their own unresolved childhood and developmental issues.

Destructive patterns affecting meaningful relationships with both self and others continue to manifest in our lives despite our spiritual beliefs and practices. As a result, increasing numbers of ministers, rabbis, sheikhs, priests, and other spiritual guides are coming to the realization that they must understand and use psychological principles to facilitate personal and spiritual development in themselves and in those they serve.

Psychologists are likewise moving away from previously held theories that religious beliefs are somehow "pathological." Researchers now confirm that spiritual conviction and practice are important factors in psychological healing. For example, recent psychological research projects have validated the healing influence of "faith in a compassionate deity." There has been an increasing amount of research supporting the beneficial effects of prayer, breathing techniques, and mantric sound practices upon the body and mind. Religious devotees and students have been practicing these exercises for thousands of years. This phenomenological research constitutes a significant body of knowledge. Rarely, however, is this research acknowledged in training programs for psychotherapists. When psychology focuses exclusively on symptoms and problems, it fails to include the numerous healing methodologies based upon ancient spiritual teachings. Wisdom traditions teach methods for healing that awaken people to their inherent value and purpose as human beings.

Many people have no sense of their intrinsic worth. Although psychological theories and methodologies have contributed in a general way to health, education, industry, and other social aspects of life, something deeper is missing. More and more, major studies are showing that the spiritual dimension is essential for human balance and well-being.

EXAMINING THE PROBLEM

In its attempt to resolve problems related to violence, addiction, and crime, government has increased regulations and controls over the population. State legislatures pass laws to enlarge police forces and to build new prisons, yet history has not demonstrated that excessive governmental controls result in any lessening of human dysfunction.

The disintegration of family life and high divorce rates seriously affect the security and well-being of our children. Addictive behaviors abound. People's daily lives are crowded with pressing responsibilities. Rushing from one responsibility to another, we are continuously stimulated by freeway noise, television, cellular phones, pagers, and e-mail messages. In the midst of this chaos, the Food and Drug Administration (FDA) suggested that 15 percent of the nation's children would be diagnosed with attention deficit hyperactivity disorder (ADHD) or related behaviors requiring the use of Ritalin by the year 2000 (DeGrande, 1998). Since that time a significant court action suit has been filed in New Jersey and California against the purveyors of Ritalin (Learning Disability Clinics, Inc., 2000).

The advent of managed care and large health management organizations (HMOs) has seriously affected the way we treat both psychological and medical needs. These powerful organizations, ever faithful to the bottom line, want quick fixes. They reflect the current psychic state of the American population. The negative impact of these organizations on psychological healing is serious. The roots of psychological problems are deeply embedded in the nervous system and may not be resolved in twelve or twenty sessions, or any specific number of sessions set by HMOs. Many psychiatrists readily prescribe psychotropic drugs. People take them hoping for a quick fix, but will these psychopharmaceutical drugs resolve our current problems? Is the prevailing biologically based medical model wrong—or a myth?

Existential psychologist Rollo May described myths as narrative patterns giving significance and meaning to our existence. He believes the dilemma in this postmodern age is an absence of currently meaningful mythology (Dossey, 1991; May, 1991). Many people today experience a total absence of meaning in their troubled lives. They cannot meet the expectations of being a "perfect machine" or performing with the cognitive accuracy demanded of computers. Existential anxiety has intensified, and medications, while often helpful in the short term, are not an absolute solution. People need to know that they are more than a problem needing to be fixed or a diagnosis to be treated. Psychotropic medications are helpful for those who experience extreme states of anxiety and depression. Far too many physicians view these drugs as cure-alls, and take little time or interest in the "circumstances" impacting their clients' feeling states.

Frequently, pharmaceutical drugs for depression and/or anxiety provide relief for a few months, and then suddenly a wave of non-integrated emotions "pushes through" the chemical barrier. Depression and anxiety are signs announcing that something in one's life or unconscious is being neglected or is unresolved. The affective message can also be the voice of the rejected aspect of the psyche demanding attention. Unfortunately, a traditional psychiatrist will often simply increase the dosage or attempt a new combination of drugs.

The biological-medical model of psychiatric illness encourages its practitioners to blame the body for serious psychological difficulties and to control this condition through the use of psychotropic medications. For example, there were approximately thirty-five advertisements for psychopharmaceutical drugs before the published articles began in the July 1997 edition of *The American Journal of Psychiatry,* published by the American Psychiatric Association. Readers were told in these ads that Paxil can lift depression and relive associated anxiety symptoms and also that it alleviates panic and obsessive-compulsive disorders.

A large ad for Effexor, an antidepressant, displayed a photo of two happy women hugging each other. Alongside that image was an open journal, with a rose resting on it and handwritten words in the journal: "I got my friend back." The ad announced to the reader that Effexor not only alleviated sadness and depression (and resolved social isolation) but was also able to treat and relieve the complications of fear.

Many people seem to have forgotten the inherent meaning of life. They are not using their innate capacities for discernment. The darkness that accompanies uncomfortable feelings, disturbing thoughts, and intimations of entering new life stages is avoided at all costs. The heroic journey is halted at its first step; signs promising psychospiritual growth are ignored; the state of exile is enhanced.

There is a Sufi story of the wise "fool of God," Mulla Nasruddin, that illustrates this danger (Shah, 1964, p. 77):

> One day the Mulla was thinking aloud. "How do I know whether I am dead or alive?"
>
> "Don't be such a fool," his wife said; "if you were dead your limbs would be cold."
>
> Shortly afterwards Nasruddin was in the forest cutting wood. It was midwinter. Suddenly he realized that his hands and feet were cold. "I am undoubtedly dead," he thought; "so I must stop working, because corpses do not work." And, because corpses do not walk about, he lay down on the grass.
>
> Soon a pack of wolves appeared and started to attack Nasruddin's donkey, which was tethered to a tree. "Yes, carry on, take advantage of a dead man," said Nasruddin from his prone position; "but if I had been alive I would not have allowed you to take liberties with my donkey."

Nasruddin's parable can be applied to the current medical model. Because HMOs and managed health care systems prefer that doctors medicate patients and perform shortsighted quick fixes, opportunities for psychospiritual insight and healing can be lost. Life narratives that involve struggles and initiatory processes necessary to individuation are overlooked and neatly swept under the rug. Instead, people are encouraged to take prescription drugs as a solution to anxiety or disease. These biomedical paradigms choose to ignore the many integrative healing approaches available through a variety of psychospiritual traditions—traditions that contain the potential to reunite body, mind, and spirit.

In many native cultures, a symptom of psychospiritual disturbance is often perceived as an indication that something greater is about to occur in the individual's life. Illness or psychic distress are signs that some challenge needs to be met or an ordeal undertaken. It is, simply put, a wake-up call announcing that there is something more to attend to than the mundane circumstances in one's life.

Life crises often force us into new dimensions of learning and experience. A call to individuation urges us to set upon a path of living life more fully, a path on which our personal despair offers intimations of victory and transformation. The heroic journey begins: a door opens and we enter the dark terrain of the personal and collective unconscious. If we embark upon this journey we will discover nonordinary states of consciousness and intimations of something more fulfilling than anything we have yet encountered in our ordinary egoic consciousness. A crisis of despair suddenly takes on a new meaning, and limiting self-narratives are reframed as the journey unfolds. The symptoms of distress become signposts along the journey. The poetry of Kabir offers an illuminating view of depression (Bly, 1977, p. 1),

> When my friend is away from me, I am
> depressed;
> nothing in the daylight delights me,
> sleep at night gives no rest,
> who can I tell about this?
>
> The night is dark, and long . . . hours go by . . .
> because I am alone, I sit up suddenly,
> fear goes through me . . .
>
> Kabir says: Listen, my friend
> there is one thing in the world that satisfies,
> and that is a meeting with the Guest.

Kabir lets us know that depression, loneliness, and fear can be evidence of longing for spiritual unity.

Existential psychologists emphasize finding "meaning" in our anxiety, difficult emotional states, and life circumstances. Each moment is a valid part of the human experience. Archetypal psychologists also suggest that feelings of depression, sorrow, and rage are soulic expressions to be lived with and appreciated—their poetical force can enrich consciousness. Learning to be a friend to feelings deepens the character, gives soul to the personality, and opens us to frequencies and experiences outside of the egoic-cognitive mind (Gilligan, 1997).

When an individual experiences depression or psychic crisis in a psychospiritually oriented community, he or she is not placed in a diagnostic category based upon a pathological view of human experience. Difficult psychospiritual experiences are believed to be passages associated with spiritual awakening, rebirth, and transformation, and are tended as such by the community.

Psychological symptoms can be viewed as signposts reminding us of unfinished personal work. Perhaps we have not paid proper attention to those parts of ourselves that dwell below the threshold of consciousness. These often conflicted and unheard voices demand attention. Clearly, our external relationships mirror our intrapsychic world. Our psychospiritual work includes listening to, learning from, and healing our wounded, unresolved, and incomplete feelings.

For twenty years I pondered my life mission. What was I born to do? Throughout this time I struggled with relational difficulties with both self and others. This struggle was rooted in identity crises related to early life experiences. Finally I came to the understanding that my "life mission" was uniquely revealed in the circumstances and healing work related to my childhood. The plot had been carefully laid down. It was my work to complete the story, cherishing and attending to each detail as thoroughly as possible. Today when clients or friends bring up questions concerning their life work, I first examine the warp and weft of their life experiences. Then I ask: "What is the meaning of our human existence? Is it to live on the surface of life and compromise our dreams, or to become the truest, most authentic human being possible?" This is where spirituality and psychology meet.

The "sacred marriage" of psychology and spirituality encourages us to experience healing across a wider spectrum and deeper range than that afforded by either discipline alone. Psychospirituality is a holistic paradigm patterned upon principles of universality and inclusion. As we integrate psychology and spirituality, our perspective shifts from one of trying to repair a dysfunctional machine to one of recognizing the inherent value of human nature and experience.

This book illustrates many of the integrative healing practices found in the world's religious and spiritual traditions. It is intended for practitioners of psychotherapy, religious counselors, and students of religious studies. It is not a book about dogma, nor is it intended to promote one religion over another. In the field of psychology we learn that certain types of therapies work better for some than for others. A good psychotherapist recognizes this and is able to change his or her therapeutic approach, or to refer a client to a more appropriate psychotherapist. Each human being is a unique creation influenced by a combination of varied life experiences. It doesn't make sense that one method should apply to all equally. Humanistic schools of psychotherapy teach their practitioners to listen—truly listen—to their clients. When we learn to listen for the nuances and depths in people, we can respond appropriately and effectively.

The practitioner of psychospirituality does not need to use his or her own religious beliefs to unduly influence persons seeking help. If experience and intuition suggest that a specific teaching or practice might be appropriate for a student or a client to consider, then we can share it in that spirit. The goal is not one of indoctrination but one of assistance. Persons sharing spiritually oriented practices should have both personal experience and qualified training.

THE SHADOW SIDE OF NEGLECT

Unfortunately, many spiritual leaders have failed to properly represent their religious ideals. They have abused their followers mentally, emotionally, and sometimes physically or sexually. Their "enlightened state" did not seem to have any effect upon the immature personality forces moving within them. This is one of the problems which results from a spirituality that negates the psychology of human experience, encouraging dualism. Our human feelings and experiences are valid expressions of life. It is emotional carelessness and dishonesty that manifest in abuse. We can never neglect the psychological work accompanying true spiritual transformation. If we are stuck in our heads or out of touch with our bodies, the active forces within our bodies are neglected—"the right hand doesn't know what the left hand is doing."

It is also a well-known fact that a number of psychotherapists have sexually abused their clients or have otherwise taken advantage of them. Perhaps these psychotherapists failed to apply in-depth psychotherapeutic work in their own lives. Perhaps in some cases they ignored spiritual influences that could have prevented unwise and predatory behaviors. The ability to truly help others requires a strong character and an evolved outlook. Such traits as a keen sensitivity, intuition, creativity, integrity, knowledge of one's field, along with compassion and wisdom, greatly assist the helping professions. It is not easy to live up to these many important qualities. Too many spiritual and psychological authority figures assume that they have "arrived" and forget that the cultivation of these traits is a lifetime endeavor.

Equally disturbing is a tendency for "new age" practitioners to take a workshop or training course, read a few books, and then "open for business." This is more than just false advertising; the in-depth inner and outer training and character development required to be exemplars and teachers is a sacred trust. It takes highly focused personal dedication, sacrifice, compassion, and self-mastery to manifest the realities of a true new age. The practices shared within the following chapters are examples of practices used by qualified and trained teachers.

INTEGRATING SCIENCE AND RELIGION

Many psychotherapy clients say that "talk therapy" failed to help them. They are seeking something deeper, and they respond to experiential psychotherapies. Also, many persons are no longer willing to settle for passive acceptance of religious theology. They want meaningful experience. There has been increasing interest in experiential spiritual practices found in various forms of contemplative prayer and meditation, Yoga, Native American and shamanic ritual, Eastern and Middle Eastern (Sufi) mantric sound and breath practices in the past few decades. Increasing numbers of people are choosing processes that expand and deepen consciousness because they offer a more direct, positive, and integrated psychospiritual experience. These processes facilitate healing and growth, enlarging and enhancing a person's previously limited identity.

The wisdom practices found in the world's spiritual traditions can guide us through internal and external difficulties. Many poets, mystics, saints, and prophets have left virtual maps to illuminate the heroic journey. Psychotherapists and students of religious studies benefit from their contributions. Psychospiritual models of healing view crisis as an opportunity for development of the soul and character.

Allusions to heroic journeys manifest repeatedly in myth and religion, from the Epic of Gilgamesh and the hymns to the Goddess Inanna (third millennium B.C.E) to the stories of the lives of Moses, Krishna, Buddha, Jesus, and Muhammad. Each one embarked on a dangerous journey or was exiled from the land of their birth (Campbell, 1949, 1974). Obstacles and opposition confronted them but each one returned a victor and made a contribution to humankind. Their messages have resounded through the ages. Why? Because they touch our souls and illuminate what appears to be a pattern inherent in the human experience. Difficult passages in life become occasions of transformation and healing, giving positive meaning to our emotional, mental, and situational disturbances.

This book demonstrates the need for a renewed tradition of psychology and spirituality. The following chapters reveal that psychospirituality is really a new term for a very old paradigm, encompassing both psychological and spiritual understanding. To foster a resurgence of psychospirituality, I have selectively gathered the estimable contributions of the authors of this anthology. Each writer has gone through years of educational training and personal experience. The chapter authors have also made significant contributions within their own traditions and fields, and to the world at large.

Readers will discover a variety of perspectives and practices used in the world's wisdom traditions in the following chapters. Each chapter will present a unique and distinctive view of psychospiritual practice and experience and demonstrate its healing applications.

Psychological training and practice needs to include the larger vistas of the soul. Such an expanded view allows us to see that human difficulties are a necessary part of the heroic journey alluded to in the world's sacred texts, mythologies, and spiritual epics. These tales tell us of the essential unity of the human and the divine. They tell us that the search for our own souls is the supreme undertaking.

REFERENCES

Bly, R. (translated) (1977). *The Kabir Book*. Boston: Beacon Press.

Campbell, J. (1949). *The Hero with a Thousand Faces*. Princeton, NJ: Princeton University Press.

Campbell, J. (1974). *The Mythic Image.* Princeton, NJ: Princeton University Press.

DeGrandre, R. (1998). *Ritalin Nation.* New York: W.W. Norton and Company.

Dossey, L. (1991). *Meaning and Medicine.* New York: Bantam Books.

Gallup Organization (1997). *The Gallup Poll: Public Opinion 1996.* Wilmington, DE: Scholastic Resources, Inc.

Gilligan, S. (1997). *The Courage to Love.* New York: W.W. Norton and Company.

Learning Disability Clinics, Inc. (2000). *Class Action Suit Against Purveyors of Ritalin.* Available online: <http://www.excelcenters.net/articles/class_action_ suit_filed.htm>. Accessed September 14, 2000.

May, R. (1991). *The Cry for Myth.* New York: W.W. Norton and Company.

Shah, I. (1964). *The Sufis.* New York: Doubleday.

The World Almanac and Book of Facts 1997 (1996). Mahwah, NJ: K-III Reference Corporation.

BUDDHISM

Buddha is your mind
And the Way goes nowhere.
Don't look for anything but this.
If you point your cart north
When you want to go south,
How will you arrive?

Buddhism is a way of life that is concerned with helping the practitioner become free of suffering through attainment of enlightenment. *Ryokan*'s (Steven, 1981, p. 56) words suggest the preciousness of the present moment. Enlightenment is not found somewhere else—in another place or time—rather it is found right here, right now.

There are many Buddhist parables concerning the quest for enlightenment. In *Zen Flesh, Zen Bones* Paul Reps and Nyogen Senzaki (1957) share a parable titled "Open Your Treasure House." Similar to many Buddhist parables it begins with the student asking the master to point the way. It illustrates the idea that the enlightened mind is already present if we can but recognize it. Even the search for enlightenment is itself a manifestation of our enlightened nature.

There are many forms of Buddhism including the Hinayana, Mahayana, and Vajrayana schools. Each one emphasizes training in mindfulness and awareness. The Buddhist practitioner works to free the mind from dualistic views to realize the inherent interdependence of all life in each moment. Each individual school has also cultivated specific strengths. For example, the Hinayana tradition emphasizes self-discipline, self-liberation, effort, and responsibility. The Mahayana stresses compassion, openness, and benefiting others. It emphasizes the *bodhisattva* vow of liberating all life from unenlightened bondage. The *bodhisattva* is an enlightened being that chooses to remain with all life until everything has known enlightenment. The Vajrayana method focuses on transcending both positive and negative elements to benefit both the individual and the world.

Buddhist psychology has much to offer the Western world. Very few persons live fully engaged in the present moment. A friend comes to visit, but the visit is continually interrupted as the friend answers pager messages. In cars, stores, workshops, and airports, people talk on cellular phones. We are fragmented people living in a fragmented society. Buddhism teaches mindfulness. Its practitioner learns to be present in each moment, thought, feeling, and movement.

In Chapter 1, Dr. Wegela presents the basic principles of contemplative psychotherapy, a Buddhist-based approach to helping clients develop mindfulness, *maitri,* and a sense of path. The teachings are based on the method of contemplative psychotherapy as it is taught and practiced at Naropa University in Boulder, Colorado, one of the first institutions to develop a program interfacing psychotherapy and Buddhism. Its roots are in the Tibetan Vajrayana tradition.

Dr. Wegela discusses, with clinical examples, the importance of cultivating genuine relationships and the notion that even seemingly mindless behaviors may be utilized in helping people to work with anxiety and other common psychological complaints. This expression of Buddhism offers us a path that returns us to what contemplative psychologists call "brilliant sanity."

Chapter 1

Nurturing the Seeds of Sanity: A Buddhist Approach to Psychotherapy

Karen Kissel Wegela

Dennis is playing third base. He is speaking softly and vehemently. On the sidelines, we can't quite hear what he is saying. He gestures with his hands and arms, waving them in wide circles as he speaks. The lines in his brow become furrowed as he appears to concentrate on what he is hearing. He is conversing with someone none of the rest of us can see or hear. The batter hits the ball; it soars upward. Dennis is ready; he is positioned under the ball, and he makes a clean catch. He throws it neatly to the pitcher. The other team has one out. Soon, Dennis resumes his private conversation.

In conventional terminology, Dennis is having vivid hallucinations. He was diagnosed many years ago with a psychotic disorder, and there is little question that he spends most of his time in a private world that is inaccessible to others. He is often terrified by what his internal voices tell him. What, then, is going on when he plays baseball? He is quite able to handle the demands of the game appropriately. He can drop his private conversation and be fully present with the details of the game as it unfolds. The incident described happened when Dennis was trying out for a local intramural team; the team did not accept him. His "weirdness" was all too obvious.

What was less obvious was the sanity that is never too far away and was revealed by his precise attentiveness to the batter, the ball, and the other demands of the game. In contemplative psychotherapy, which is based on Buddhist teachings, we are always looking for ways to nurture the seeds of sanity which may be found in even the most confused states of mind (Podvoll, 1990).

INTRODUCTION

More than 2,500 years ago, the man we have come to call the Buddha, which means "Awakened One," taught that both the causes of our suffering and the path to freedom from that suffering lie within ourselves. The approach to psychotherapy known as contemplative psychotherapy, developed and taught at the Naropa University (formerly The Naropa Institute) in Boulder, Colorado, since 1975, joins together the teachings of Buddhism and the Western tradition of psychotherapy.

Contemplative psychotherapy teaches that to be fully human, and to discover the sanity within each of us, we need to develop mindfulness and awareness. In the Buddhist path this is done primarily through various meditative practices. In contemplative psychotherapy we help clients develop mindfulness and awareness not by requiring them to meditate, but through the therapeutic relationship itself and by working with the activities of their everyday lives.

In this chapter we will examine some basic Buddhist teachings and explore their applications in contemplative psychotherapy. In all of the clinical examples provided details have been changed to protect the privacy of clients. Because contemplative psychotherapy and Buddhism emphasize being awake to our experience in the present moment, let us begin with two experiential exercises. These exercises may provide a reference point for some of the following discussion.

Experiential Exercise 1: Mindfulness Practice

> First, one takes a good posture sitting in a chair or on a cushion on the floor. One sits upright, straight but not rigid. The eyes remain open, and the gaze rests on the floor about four to six feet away. The breathing is natural. Now, for five minutes or so, one simply notices the experience of breathing. If one's mind wanders away from noticing the breathing, one gently returns to paying attention to it. After five minutes, one reflects on what one experienced.

Most people find that their minds wander away quite readily. Even if they try very hard to stay focused on their breathing, it is likely that they will find themselves lost in thoughts and fantasies or caught up with physical or emotional feelings. This is not a problem, but it reveals how difficult it is to simply be present and mindful.

In the next exercise, instead of trying to be mindful, the meditator seeks to experience mindlessness.

Experiential Exercise 2: Mindlessness Practice

The meditator adjusts the posture, eye gaze, breathing, and mind to become as "absent" as possible. If one wanders into being present, he or she returns gently to the practice of mindlessness. Again, the practitioner takes about five minutes to do this exercise and then reflects back on what was experienced.

Most people find this exercise much easier to do than Exercise 1. They have little trouble becoming lost in thoughts and worries, enjoying a good sensual fantasy, spacing out into a dulled state, or losing track of where they are with their racing thoughts.

These exercises are important because contemplative psychotherapy uses both our human capacity for mindfulness and our talent for mindlessness in working with others. We will look at this more later in the chapter, but first let us turn to some basic teachings common to Buddhism and contemplative psychotherapy.

Since the time of the Buddha, a great many different Buddhist schools have developed. Although their basic teachings, known as the Dharma, tend to agree, they have very different styles—from the austerity of the Japanese Zen schools to the elaborate and colorful rituals of the Tibetan Vajrayana. Given this variety, it is not surprising that it is traditional to identify one's lineage and one's teachers. My own main teacher was Chögyam Trungpa Rinpoche, a master in the Kagyu and Nyingma schools of Tibetan Buddhism. He founded the Naropa University in 1974 as a place where the teachings of the West and the East could encounter each other. The explanations that follow are based largely on my study with him and others in the Kagyu and Nyingma schools, and any errors contained herein are my own.

A key teaching in Buddhism asks us to accept nothing on faith and instead to investigate for ourselves whether or not these teachings accurately reflect our experiences.

BRILLIANT SANITY AND BUDDHA NATURE

In contemplative psychotherapy we use the term *brilliant sanity* to refer to our most fundamental nature. In some schools of Buddhism this is called *Buddha nature* or *tathagatagarbha* (Maitreya and Asanga, 1985).

It is quite difficult to describe brilliant sanity in words because it is not conceptual, but I'll try to describe it. Often when we've been surprised, pleasantly or unpleasantly, we are able to experience phenomena without the filters of language, expectation, or bias. Our habits of perception have been temporarily suspended, and we glimpse brilliant sanity.

An Example: Brilliant Sanity

A week ago I was in a minor car accident. I was struck from behind as I waited to make a turn. My car lurched into the one in front of me. I had a momentary image of airbags that hadn't deployed, a physical sense of being jolted, and it was over. A moment of stillness followed. Then, with my mind quite slowed down, I looked up to see a woman in a bright red cable-knit sweater making her way over the icy road toward me. As I got out of my car I could feel the chilly air on my cheeks, the wind whipping my hair around, and the trembling that was occurring all over my body.

The next moment the red-sweatered lady was giving me a big hug. She was warm and earthy, and her dark hair danced in the wind. I turned around and noticed a young man emerging from the truck behind me. He was moving slowly. I asked if he wanted a hug too, and he grinned shyly and said, "Oh yeah!"

As he and I hugged, enveloping each other in puffy winter jackets, the woman who had hugged me joined us. The three of us stood, a knot of humanity, hugging by the side of a busy road.

Whatever the three of us had had on our minds before the accident, we had dropped these thoughts completely. We were simply present and kind to one another. As the young man and I sat in my car, out of the below-zero cold weather, we confessed to each other how shaken we both were.

It didn't take long, of course, before we found our ways back into our habitual patterns. The red-sweatered woman left quickly since her car had no damage, and she had an engagement. I climbed comfortably into my familiar role as teacher and told the young man what we needed to do. The young man, who I suspect was a college student, gracefully played the role of one who needed to be told.

Yet we three had connected genuinely with one another: beyond any roles or differences in age, race, or affluence. What we had in common was much deeper: we had all shared brilliant sanity, Buddha nature.

Brilliant sanity has three qualities: openness, clarity, and compassion (Wegela, 1996). Openness refers to a quality of indestructible spaciousness in the mind. All of our experiences—sensations, emotions, thoughts, images—arise in the open space of the mind. It is possible to be in touch with this aspect of experience regardless of what is arising. In the moments following the accident, the sense of slowing down and simply being present with what was happening were reflections of this quality of openness.

The second quality is clarity, the ability to be precisely mindful and aware of whatever experiences we have. It is not the same as being objectively accurate, but instead refers to our capacity for direct experience. As I stood outside the car after the accident, there was an unmediated quality to my experience of the cold and the wind, which was not overlaid with thoughts or preferences.

The third quality is compassion. From this point of view, compassion, the desire to relieve unnecessary suffering, is inherent in us; it is part of our most fundamental nature. The connection that the three of us felt, hugging by the roadside, was an expression of that interconnectedness and compassion, which are aspects of our brilliant sanity.

Brilliant sanity is understood to be unconditional. This means that it is present, even if not fully manifested, in all people under all conditions. Dennis, despite his psychosis, has brilliant sanity. It is revealed in his clarity playing baseball. The task of the healer is to help others recognize and reconnect with their brilliant sanity.

THE FOUR NOBLE TRUTHS

One of the earliest discourses given by the Buddha revealed what are known as the Four Noble Truths (Trungpa, 1987). These set forth fundamental Buddhist teachings on the arising of suffering and the path to its cessation. The Four Noble Truths explain how we lose touch with our brilliant sanity and how we might reconnect with it. In brief, the Four Noble Truths are (1) the Truth of Suffering, (2) the Truth of the Origin of Suffering, (3) the Truth of the Cessation of Suffering, and (4) the Truth of the Path. Let us look at each of these as they apply to contemplative psychotherapy.

The First Noble Truth:
The Truth of Suffering

The First Noble Truth points to the reality that our lives are filled with suffering. Suffering is described in varying ways, but the core idea is that we tend to deny, hang on to, or push away whatever is painful in our lives. This pain might be obvious, for example, a psychotic disorder or a lack of adequate food and shelter. It might be subtler, for example, the vague disquiet most of us feel—a kind of low-level anxiety. We talk to ourselves in our minds, giving ourselves advice about how we ought to be different from how we are. We watch over our own shoulders to make sure we don't do anything too foolish or embarrassing. Whatever struggle we engage in to get away from how things are, and how we are, is regarded as suffering.

Many of the people who seek therapy do so because they are aware of pain in their lives. Often they feel that it is a sign of failure on their part. Sometimes the initial work of therapy is simply for clients to begin to acknowledge the pain they feel and to discriminate between the direct experience of pain and the judgments that have been placed on top of it.

The Buddha taught that the experience of pain is not a sign that there is anything wrong with us or proof that we are living our lives incorrectly. Rather, it is an aspect of being alive in a body. Birth, old age, sickness, and death are the traditional examples of the pain attendant in being embodied. The problem is not with the pain per se, but with our struggle against it.

The Second Noble Truth: The Truth of the Origin of Suffering

In the Second Noble Truth the Buddha points to the source of our suffering: the attempt to create and grasp a solid sense of self. We use the term *ego* in referring to this attempt to construct a sense of self, which is permanent, separate, and solid. In Buddhist teachings, and in contemplative psychotherapy, we use the term ego in this very specific way. (Other uses of this term in contemporary psychology may refer to our ability to contact our experience, to use logic, or to have confidence. Although the Buddhist teachings indicate that our struggle to create and maintain an ego is a problem, these contemporary notions of ego are not seen as problematic.)

In the Buddhist view, we can find nothing in our experience that is unchanging. It is a common Buddhist contemplation to look for something unchanging in ourselves. Our thoughts, our sensations, our emotions, our mental imagery, the very molecules and atoms that form our bodies—all of these are changing. What then, ask the Buddhists, is this permanent something which we all regard as ourselves?

We can point to a river with its constantly changing flow of water, and we might call it by the same name today and tomorrow. In the same way, we indicate ourselves and give ourselves names, but there is nothing in us that remains unchanged over time.

To regard ourselves as separate is to ignore our interconnectedness with others and all phenomena. Everything we regard as "self" is made up of what Thich Nhat Hanh, a Vietnamese Zen teacher, calls "nonself elements" (Hanh, 1990). Similar to a flower that is made up of the nonflower elements of water, sunlight, earth, and so on, our "selves" are made up of nonself elements. Our bodies are made up of interconnecting organ systems. Even our thoughts are made up of colors, shapes, and images that we have seen elsewhere. When we sit quietly in meditation, we can notice all of the images, bits of fast-food jingles, snatches of remembered conversations, and scripts of imagined future victories and so on, with which we fill our minds. All of these individual thoughts are hardly what we could call a self. Wherever we look, we find nonself elements. We are made up of a unique interconnection, in any one moment, of all these nonself elements.

We are also interconnected with each other. When I am with someone else, of what is my experience made? It includes my perceptions (and projections) of the other person (McLeod, 1989). Where is the me that is separate from my experience of the other person? Can I find one? The Buddhist would say no, I cannot. It is our interconnectedness that is reflected in natural compassion.

Finally, to say we are solid is to imply that there is something in us which cannot be broken down into smaller nonself elements. It is similar to saying that one part of the river stays in the same spot and is unaffected by the flowing water. The Buddhists ask if we can find such a solid, unchanging, indivisible something in our experience, and they suggest that we cannot.

When we try to create and cling to an ego, we are trying to do something that is impossible. The result is suffering. We tend to avoid any experience that challenges our sense of self as solid, permanent, and unchanging. For example, we try to escape feelings of uncertainty and vulnerability. In the United States we pride ourselves on being independent and constant. Yet from the Buddhist point of view we are nothing of the kind. When we experience moments of brilliant sanity—which we might at any moment because it is our true nature—we tend to respond to them by feeling anxious or irritated. We would rather continue with what is familiar, even if it is unpleasant, than open up to what is intense, vivid, and novel. This is an important idea to explore in our own experiences. We all believe we value freshness and originality, but how often do we turn away from what threatens the status quo?

Whenever we live our lives in accordance with the dictates of ego clinging, we narrow our world. We avoid situations that are at odds with the notions we have of ourselves. Often clients arrive in therapy because their senses of themselves are being challenged. A client might feel depression and lack of meaning after losing a long-held job. Rather than helping clients to patch together an impossible-to-maintain ego, a contemplative psychotherapist is likely to explore with the client how their expectations differ from what is actually happening. They might discuss how the attempt to maintain an out-of-date conception of oneself leads to problems. Instead of trying to build or support a nonexistent ego, a more realistic goal is increased flexibility.

The primary way we manage to avoid recognizing our true nature is by cultivating mindlessness. Mindlessness is cultivated by desynchronizing body and mind. Recalling the exercise at the beginning of this chapter, a great many ways can be used to attain mindlessness. Some common mindlessness practices are watching television, playing computer games, and jogging with headphones. We can cultivate mindlessness through mental activities—obsessing, worrying, spacing out, fantasizing. Similar to small children who cling to a favorite toy or blanket, we often seek security in mindlessness.

Whenever we engage in a mindlessness practice, we are being subtly, or not so subtly, self-aggressive: we are rejecting our present experience, that is, who we are in the present moment. When we cultivate self-aggression we plant the seeds not of sanity but of psychopathology (Hanh, 1990). Underneath mental distress is the belief that we are basically bad or fundamentally flawed (Wegela and Joseph, 1992). This is, of course, ego in another guise. In this case, the ego is supported by a story of basic unworthiness, low self-esteem, or badness. It is a variation of the subtle kind of pain in which we feel that something is somehow wrong with us. This conviction leads to further attempts to escape ourselves and to still more efforts to become mindless.

We co-opt a good deal of creativity in our cultivation of mindlessness. We are able to pervert any activity, including spiritual practices, into mindlessness practices. Instead of using meditation, mantra, yoga, or prayer to help us to connect with that which is most true or sacred, we use them to dissociate ourselves from our experience. Chögyam Trungpa Rinpoche coined the term *spiritual materialism* for this attempt to build ego through the misuse of spiritual practices (Trungpa, 1987). We might, for example, use a meditation practice as a way to avoid contact with others, or we might try to block out unpleasant emotions by repeating a mantra mindlessly to ourselves.

How can we tell when we are cultivating mindlessness? Several hallmarks can help us. When we are engaged in mindlessness practices we lose contact with our environment. We no longer notice pain or anxiety. Perhaps more telling is our response to interruption. We become irritated if anyone dares to disrupt our concentration when we are cultivating mindlessness. Instead of saying, "Thank you for waking me up," we are more apt to growl or snap.

A more important hallmark of mindlessness is our loss of compassion. Sometimes this is exactly why we cultivate mindlessness. It is very painful to feel the suffering of others, to recognize the pain, disease, and poverty that occurs all over the planet. Ironically, it is our naturally tender hearts, the compassionate nature of brilliant sanity, that leads us sometimes to seek mindlessness.

The price of cultivating mindlessness is quite high: we lose touch with brilliant sanity, and we fail to relieve the suffering of others. We feel half alive, alienated, and lonely; we suffer. We become selfish and lose track of our hearts.

One woman with whom I worked in therapy was quite gifted at disconnecting from what was happening around her. She would look present, but she was barely there. Although this had been a useful skill when she had been the victim of childhood abuse, now it was preventing her from feeling and showing love to her husband and children. When she came to therapy she said she had realized that she was missing her life. Her children regarded her as a zombie. It was palpably painful to her that she was not available to them in the way that she wanted to be.

Coming to understand how suffering is cultivated through the attempt to create ego and then maintained through practices of mindlessness is the expression of the Second Noble Truth in contemplative psychotherapy.

The Third Noble Truth:
The Truth of the Cessation of Suffering

The Third Noble Truth states that all of this unnecessary suffering can come to an end. Traditionally, liberation or enlightenment means that one is freed from the cycle of rebirth in *samsara,* confused existence. In contemplative psychotherapy, we would say that we can reconnect with brilliant sanity: we can stop perpetuating the personal warfare involved in the self-deception of trying to create ego. We may learn how to relax into ourselves. Instead of practicing self-aggression by trying to be what we are not, we can relax our struggle and make friends with who we really are. Because it is our nature to be open, awake, and compassionate, it requires a lot of work to maintain the illusion of ego. Actually, if we bring our curiosity to the task, we may discover that we have moments and glimpses of brilliant sanity all the time. An important idea here is what is known as *maitri. Maitri* is a Sanskrit word (Pali: "Metta") that is usually translated as "loving kindness." Traditionally it means the desire for all beings to be happy.

Maitri is also used to refer to an attitude of unconditional friendliness to all aspects of one's experience. Rather than rejecting anything, we learn to develop curiosity and warmth. *Maitri* means that whatever arises in our experience, we meet it by seeing it clearly and letting it be what it is. If an experience of anxiety arises, having *maitri* toward it means simply experiencing the trembling, fear, and mental imagery that accompany the experience. It is the absence of struggle. In the same way that good friends continue to love us despite our flaws, having *maitri* means that we do not reject ourselves or any parts of our experience.

There are a number of ways we might misunderstand the notion of *maitri.* First, having *maitri* is not the same thing as liking something. To like something is to have judged it. We don't have to like the experience of anxiety to have *maitri* toward it.

Second, *maitri* is not "being nice" to oneself. I have heard students describe zoning out in front of the television or getting high on marijuana as "being nice" to themselves. *Maitri* is the willingness to let our experience be just what it is without trying to escape from it. It contains a quality of warmth because when we go toward our experience, we find tenderness.

Third, *maitri* is not the self-deception of saying to ourselves that everything is "all right" when we are being aggressive to ourselves or to others. Letting things be what they are means dropping self-deception. We might decide to take some kind of action, but we can't know what to do if we're not willing to see the truth of the situation first. *Maitri* is not an excuse for cowardice.

One of the subtlest ways that we might misunderstand *maitri* is to condemn ourselves for not having enough of it. We say something absurd, such as, "If I only had enough maitri, I wouldn't be so miserable." This is the activity of self-aggression, the opposite of *maitri,* which is nonaggression.

The Three Marks of Existence

Another outcome of the Buddhist spiritual path is the discovery of the Three Marks of Existence. Briefly, these are some of the aspects of our lives that are revealed when we develop mindfulness and awareness.

The first mark is impermanence. We are no longer confused about the truth of impermanence in all aspects of our being and in the phenomenal world. Since trying to create a permanent sense of self is the source of our suffering, this is an important insight. The second mark of existence is egolessness. Cessation of suffering has to do with the recognition that our true state is one of egolessness, of being without ego. Sometimes people find this idea outrageous and even frightening. Egolessness doesn't mean that there is no continuity of being; it means that nothing is solid, separate, and permanent in us. When we drop the attempt to create ego, we discover flexibility, responsiveness, and freedom. The third mark of existence is suffering. We discover that when we try to avoid impermanence and egolessness, we suffer. This mark also points, as does the First Noble Truth, to the reality of pain in our lives. The struggle to deny pain creates still more pain. Enlightenment is not about escaping from pain; it is about an end to the unnecessary suffering that we create ourselves.

The Third Noble Truth is sometimes called the Truth of the Goal. In contemplative psychotherapy our goal is to help clients reconnect with their brilliant sanity. I usually think of this as helping clients develop mindfulness and *maitri*. We will look more closely at the development of mindfulness next.

When clients have developed *maitri,* they are well on their way toward concluding their therapeutic work. Because, in the contemplative view, the ground of psychopathology is self-aggression—conviction in one's own basic badness—*maitri* is often a sign that clients have let go of that conviction. Of course, this is a gradual process, but indications of developing *maitri* are very important signposts on the path toward reconnecting with brilliant sanity.

The Fourth Noble Truth:
The Truth of the Path

The path is the method in the Buddhist spiritual journey for attaining the goal. The path is understood to require commitment to awakening, and it is regarded as something that takes a long time. Even if one does not subscribe to the idea of rebirth, the notion of gradual development is important. In American culture we often fall into a "quick fix" mentality.

The traditional description of the Buddhist approach is the *Eightfold Path* (Karthar, 1992). It is beyond the scope of this chapter to describe it in detail, but the heart of it is the cultivation of mindfulness and awareness in all the activities of one's life: the actions of body, of speech, and of mind. The idea of the path does not mean that there is a road laid out for us already, similar to the yellow brick road in *The Wizard of Oz*. Rather, each of us has to discover the true path for ourselves with the example of the Buddha, the help of our teachers, the teachings of the Dharma, and the community of fellow practitioners (the *sangha*). Still, we are on our own, and part of the journey lies in recognizing the paradox that although we are interconnected, we are still alone.

The various teachings in the Eightfold Path can help us to "stay on the path" by indicating what to cultivate and from what to refrain. Most simply, the early teachings of the Buddha state that we should refrain from harming others. Later teachings, those of the Mahayana schools, say that the true path is found in attaining enlightenment for the benefit of others.

A lot of discussion and controversy currently surrounds whether psychotherapy can, in itself, provide a genuine path to awakening (Watson, Batchelor, and Claxton, 2000). My own sense is that psychotherapy may be part of such a path, but it is not enough on its own.

Part of the power of psychotherapy is that it happens in the context of human relationship. In the Buddhist tradition, an important aspect of the path is working with being alone. One learns to take responsibility for one's own state of mind. It is easy to become dependent upon a therapist and lose track of this important insight. Moreover, a spiritual journey, especially a meditative discipline, is a lifelong commitment. Psychotherapy may be a stage in the journey, but it is not usual for it to become a lifelong endeavor.

Clients come to psychotherapy for many reasons. Often they come because they are experiencing personal crises that are reflections of the three marks of existence. They might, for example, realize that they are not who they thought they were due to the loss of a relationship or the onset of an illness. They might be having trouble relating to the reality of impermanence: for example, they are growing older or they are grieving the loss of loved ones. More simply, they may be suffering from the pain of depression or anxiety.

At other times clients enter therapy because they have lost the sense of path in their lives or have never had one. They are not sure what is important to them, and they have no basis for making meaningful decisions about how to proceed. Helping clients discover, or rediscover, this quality is often a significant part of their work in therapy.

Accepting the idea of a gradual path is often a reflection of developing *maitri*. Instead of self-aggressively demanding that they change immediately, clients become more at home with themselves. This leads to softening, relaxation, and *maitri*.

THE PATH OF CONTEMPLATIVE PSYCHOTHERAPY

This section looks at two important aspects of the work of helping clients reconnect with their brilliant sanity: the development of genuine relationship and the cultivation of mindfulness.

One of the working assumptions in contemplative psychotherapy is the need for a genuine relationship between the therapist and the client. It is a specialized relationship in that it focuses primarily on the client's concerns. However, the therapist must have the ability to be present as fully as possible and the willingness to experience directly the intensity provoked in him or her by the client's experience.

Shamatha/Vipashyana *Sitting Practice*

Shamatha/vipashyana—mindfulness/awareness sitting meditation (see Photo 1.1)—is an essential part of the training and ongoing discipline of all contemplative psychotherapists. If therapists are to assist clients in nurturing the seeds of their basic sanity, they must be intimately familiar with their own patterns of turning away from brilliant sanity.

Therapists need to work through and let go of their own ego-driven stories, biases, and expectations, which are the basis of countertransference. An ongoing mindfulness/awareness practice provides this. It is not my intention to provide meditation instruction here, but I will note that the practice we teach students as Naropa involves learning to discriminate between being present and not being present. It provides the opportunity to become very familiar with one's own patterns of leaving the present moment by trying to create ego.

Moreover, because the technique itself contains an alternation of touching one's experience and letting it go, the practice of mindfulness/awareness meditation allows one to become comfortable with space: uncertainty, confusion, and the absence of story.

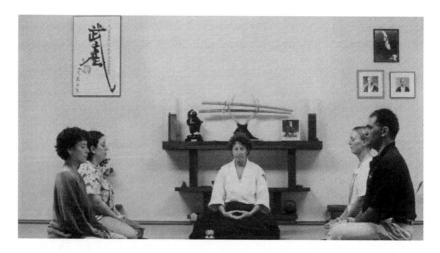

PHOTO 1.1. "Sitting meditation by Zen practitioners." Courtesy of Sensei Coryl Crane and North County Aikikai, Solana Beach, California.

Tonglen *Practice*

A second practice in which contemplative psychotherapists engage is *tonglen,* a Mahayana practice that cultivates compassion (Chodron, 1994). The ground (basis) of this practice is recognizing the spaciousness and warmth of our nature. Given this "emptiness" and compassion, we are able to practice taking in the pain of others and breathing out to them relief from their suffering. Contemplative psychotherapists practice *tonglen* "on the cushion" (in their formal meditation practice) and also on the spot with their clients.

Maitri *Space Awareness Practice*

One last practice, which is part of the training of contemplative psychotherapists, is *maitri* space awareness. In Naropa training, this practice is done in the context of a residential retreat community and in conjunction with sitting practice. It involves holding specific postures, derived from Tibetan yoga, in specially designed rooms of five different shapes and colors. Each room evokes different states of mind in the practitioner. The practice is based on the five Buddha families, which correspond to five elemental energies: space, water, earth, fire, and wind (Trungpa, 1987). Each one is associated with particular personality styles, both neurotic and sane. The *vajra* family, for example, is associated with water, winter, dawn, and the East. Its neurotic aspect is aggression or anger, and its sane aspect is called *mirrorlike wisdom.* Everyone's experience in each room is personal and unique, yet it is quite common for people to have variations of these experiences. The basic energy of the neurotic and sane aspects is the same. The neurotic manifestation is the result of trying to reference the experience of mirrorlike wisdom, or clarity, to ego. To reject our experience, i.e., to be aggressive or angry, we first have to glimpse it clearly. Only then can we react by pushing it away because we don't like it or it doesn't fit our sense of ourselves.

Doing this practice in the context of a community of practitioners gives one the opportunity to have oneself mirrored back. The members of the community also engage in the ordinary activities of keeping the community running: cooking, cleaning, etc. As one might imagine, the chances to come into conflict and to receive support and feedback are myriad.

Being a member of a *maitri* community leads to several possible discoveries. First, practitioners discover that they are not only who they thought they were. Nearly everyone finds that they feel quite different as they rotate through the five rooms. This does a good job of experientially pointing out egolessness.

The *maitri* practice often helps students to become acquainted with and relax with intensity. The rooms provoke intense states of mind for many. For psychotherapists in training this is very important. If we are not at home with intensity, we will tend to abort our clients' experiences of intensity.

In contemplative psychotherapy we use the term *therapeutic aggression* to refer to any attempt on the therapist's part to get the client to change so that the therapist can feel more comfortable or competent (Fortuna, 1987). *Maitri* space awareness practice is very helpful in preparing us to see and let go of this common tendency.

Another important aspect of the *maitri* training is that it helps students to recognize sanity in all of its many disguises. Just as there is clarity to be found in anger, all of the Buddha families point to the hidden wisdoms to be found in neurotic emotions.

The Phenomenon of Exchange

In contemplative psychotherapy we use the word "exchange" to refer to our direct experience of another person (Wegela, 1988). Exchange is different from countertransference, which is our reaction to another based on our own history. Exchange is a direct experience in the present moment not referenced to anything else.

I met once with a woman about whom I knew very little. I noticed that my mind was starting to feel as though it had jangling and loud electrical pulsations in it. My thoughts were coming with increasing rapidity, and my jaw began to feel tight. As we continued to talk, it became clear that this woman was in the early stages of a psychotic episode. The experiences I had were not simply a reaction to her; they were similar to what she was experiencing herself.

It is important to note that we filter our experiences of exchange in the same way we do anything else. Unless we are enlightened and constantly in touch with brilliant sanity, we tend to filter experiences through our expectations, memories, and biases.

Exchange is ongoing; it is not a technique but a naturally occurring phenomenon that reflects our interconnectedness. It is very useful for therapists to learn to think in terms of it. We always hold tentatively any ideas we have about exchange because ego can be very subtle.

When we have a sense of what someone else's experience is, we can feel more compassion. If, instead, we pull back from the exchange, we are not likely to be very helpful.

The Technique of "Touch and Go"

The technique we use to work with exchange comes from sitting practice: touch and go (Wegela, 1988). As part of our practice discipline, we learn to momentarily, but completely, touch our experience as it arises. For example, a moment of rage may be felt in the body with its accompanying energy, mental imagery, and words. In the next moment, we let it go again. Another way to say this is that we allow it to go, without trying to manipulate it any further. Since all of the elements of our experience are impermanent, they are always changing. Unless we hang on to them, they will go. Letting go can also be regarded as "letting be." The idea is that there is a rhythm of going toward our experience and then relaxing.

Contemplative psychotherapists practice touch and go in working with exchange. This is a practical method for being present and not getting lost. Sometimes, of course, we all get lost. When we notice we are lost, we simply and gently return to practicing touch and go.

As we sit with our clients working with touch and go, we bring two important qualities into our experience: mindfulness and *maitri*. In touching we bring precise attention to what arises (mindfulness) and in letting go, we allow it to be what it is *(maitri)*. What happens when we practice this way can be quite powerful for the client. The client may exchange with what we are experiencing. Exchange goes both ways.

Sometimes clients' introduction to *maitri* is simply what they experience when they are with another person, perhaps a therapist, who is experiencing it on the spot. I suspect that often this is the most healing aspect of what we do. When therapists practice mindfulness and maitri, bringing precision and warmth to their own experiences and to the exchange, they affect the atmosphere of the relationship.

This may sound a bit like hocus-pocus, so I encourage readers to explore this for themselves. If we are not aware of exchange we might easily misinterpret what is happening. For example, I once began to feel frightened with a client. I might have concluded that the client was scaring me by being threatening or dangerous. However, it could be exchange. The client might have been feeling frightened himself.

Working with exchange in this way is a powerful practice for the therapist: doing psychotherapy becomes a mindfulness practice in itself. In contemplative psychotherapy we use the term *mutual recovery* to point to the idea that both the therapist and the client benefit from their work together (Podvoll, 1990).

CULTIVATING MINDFULNESS

Most kinds of psychotherapy teach some kind of mindfulness to clients. Clients learn to track their thoughts in cognitive therapy, to be precise with their dreams in Jungian work, and so on. In contemplative psychotherapy we are interested in helping clients to track the moment-to-moment occurrence of their experiences in the present. As we develop mindfulness, we can then take this skill into the rest of our lives. As mindfulness increases, we begin to see recurrent patterns. When we see how one thing leads to another, we can try different behaviors. Then we once again apply our mindfulness to noticing what we experience, having tried a new approach.

Moreover, in contemplative work, mindfulness can lead to the discovery of space and emptiness. Instead of trying to fill the space of mind with ego and its stories, we might learn to rest in the stillness that is also part of our experience instead of regarding it as a problem or proof that we are boring. Mindfulness helps us recognize that our stories about ourselves are not really solid. There is space within them and also all around them.

Another important quality of mindfulness is that it actually transforms experience. Whenever we mindlessly perpetuate ego activity and its attendant emotions and mental states, we plant the seeds of further ego activity. A discussion that would fill many pages concerns the eight kinds of consciousness, but the relevant point is that each time we experience something, we plant seeds in the deepest layers of our being for its recurrence (Hanh, 1990).

If we join mindfulness with our experience, we plant seeds of mindfulness. This is one reason why repeatedly revisiting memories of past abuse, for example, would not be regarded as a good idea from a Buddhist point of view. Unless we can bring something different to our present experience of a memory, like mindfulness or *maitri* or compassion, we will simply plant more seeds of its recurrence. In contemplative psychotherapy we make use of our clients' everyday activities to help them cultivate mindfulness.

THE FOUR FOUNDATIONS OF MINDFULNESS

A teaching common to all schools of Buddhism comes from an early *sutra,* or discourse, by the Buddha, and is known as the Four Foundations of Mindfulness (Trungpa, 1991). The Four Foundations are descriptions of the most fundamental objects to which we may apply our mindful attention. The descriptions vary from school to school, and here I will again be drawing on the oral tradition of Tibet as presented by Chögyam Trungpa Rinpoche. As he presents them, the four foundations are (1) Body, (2) Life, (3) Effort, and (4) Mind. For the contemplative psychotherapist, the Four Foundations provide a way of determining whether a particular activity is one which promotes mindfulness.

In psychotherapeutic work, we help clients to recognize bodily experiences. Mindlessness is the result of body and mind not being together, so it is especially valuable to develop Mindfulness of Body, the first foundation, and awareness of the changing sensations and perceptions of the body. This brings body and mind together.

The second foundation, Mindfulness of Life, works with the textures of life itself. The technique of touch and go is associated with this foundation and provides a method for directly experiencing the "feel" of our lives. In addition, this foundation works with our tendency to grasp on to experiences, especially any experiences that we might regard as "spiritual" or good. Instead, we learn to touch them and then to let go. When we practice in this way, we are present for each moment, not holding on to some imagined perfect state. It helps us to avoid spiritual materialism, and it undermines the tendency to cling to ego.

The third foundation, Mindfulness of Effort, is somewhat paradoxical. We usually think of effort as trying. In this foundation, however, we experience mindfulness by letting go of effort. The idea is that we return naturally to the present moment again and again. The technique associated with this foundation is the *abstract watcher.* We notice that we are back, as though there was a watcher in us. The point is that watching is not the same as judging. We note simply that we are back, without further judgment about it being bad that we were gone. This foundation points to the important notion that we must hold our minds not too tight and not too loose.

Sometimes the moment of returning to the present, free from thoughts, is experienced as a gap, an interruption in a mindless flow of words. To the extent that we try to maintain a solid sense of self, we might regard such moments as a problem, something to get past as quickly as possible. They represent a hole in our sense of ourselves. I might become curious with a client about what happened in such a moment. This is often a rich opportunity to explore a glimpse of openness or uncertainty. It might lead to recognition of the possibility of relaxing the tight habitual grip of ego activity.

The fourth foundation, Mindfulness of Mind, has to do with recognizing the uniqueness of each moment. In therapy, the fourth foundation can be useful in helping clients to recognize the subtle differences in the flow of their experiences. Rather than simply accepting a blanket description, such as "I feel depressed," I work with my clients to explore what that word means right now. The Four Foundations act together; a moment of true mindfulness contains all four together.

The Four Foundations provide a useful reference point for determining if an activity is likely to help us develop mindfulness. The more of the Four Foundations that are engaged, the more potential an activity has to cultivate mindfulness.

In contemplative psychotherapy, the therapeutic encounter itself often becomes an interpersonal mindfulness practice. As we have already seen, the therapist's task requires mindfulness of the details of the interaction as it unfolds, including the therapist's personal reactions and the experience of exchange. Of course, it also includes tracking what the client says and does. For the client, the therapy session is also an opportunity to develop mindfulness of the moment-to-moment unfolding of his or her experience. The therapist helps the client to notice body experience, the changing textures of emotions, the occurrence of gaps in habitual mind, and the uniqueness of each moment. Together, the therapist and client examine how these moments lead to patterns of behavior.

Because of their increasing mindfulness, clients come to see how their actions may be causing pain to themselves and to others. Such moments of recognition are delicate times (Podvoll, 1983). When we see how we are harming ourselves and others, often our reaction is self-revulsion. There is great sanity in such a moment, great clarity. The danger is that this may easily become self-aggression. With the help of their therapists, clients can use these times instead as opportunities to connect more deeply with brilliant sanity—with clarity, compassion, and openness. In contemplative psychotherapy such moments can lead to a *shift in allegiance* (Podvoll, 1983). Clients may feel inspired to commit themselves to refraining from the harmful behavior. In Buddhism, this is called renunciation.

Ordinary life activities provide another rich source of potential mindfulness practices. Almost anything may be used. Any pastime that involves the body is a good possibility. Most clients have some areas of cultivated mindfulness already in their lives, and contemplative psychotherapists will listen for these. I have worked with clients who have used cooking, applying fingernail polish, playing baseball, oil painting, and yoga, among other activities, as ways to develop mindfulness.

A young woman I worked with was able to apply the mindfulness she had developed as a rock climber to other areas of her life. When she climbed she paid careful attention to her body: this foot moves to here and that hand grips the rock just so. She was able to touch and go with the fear that would arise as she climbed high above the ground. She frequently experienced moments free from habitual thought; she might have a joyful moment of appreciating the beauty that surrounded her. The fourth foundation appeared in her ability to notice the fresh challenge of each moment.

As we talked it became clear that she knew a lot about holding her mind not too tight and not too loose. Moreover, she knew how to let go of distractions (such as her fearful thoughts) and return to the demands of the present moment. She quickly learned that she could apply this same skill to letting go of obsessive thoughts that she was experiencing about the well-being of her brother.

USING MINDLESSNESS PRACTICES MINDFULLY

One of the hallmarks of the Vajrayana tradition is to make use of all aspects of experience in the path of awakening. In contemplative psychotherapy we make use of mindlessness practices to develop mindfulness. As previously discussed, mindlessness practices rely on separating the experience of body from that of mind. In making use of them, the first step is for the therapist to be curious about mindlessness practices that the client demonstrates in the session or that the client describes.

This is the initial step for the client too: the development of curiosity. We ask clients to describe, in detail, how they go about conducting their mindlessness practices. For example, a favorite of mine to ask about is nail-biting. I ask: "When do you feel the desire to bite your nails? What's going on then? How do you know which nail to start with? Then what? How does the practice continue? How do you know when to stop? How do you feel doing it? What happens to your relationships with others when you're engaged in this practice?" Together we explore it thoroughly. I have found that it is often helpful to ask people to teach me their mindlessness practices and to identify their benefits.

Obviously, when people describe their mindlessness practices, they become less mindless about them. This begins to change the practice a little bit. Then, the person is encouraged to continue being curious. In addition, they become aware of how the practice is serving them and how it is not.

This is the first use of mindlessness practices: making them the object of mindfulness. There are two other valuable ways to take advantage of our aptitude for cultivating mindlessness: (1) we can choose to engage in them on purpose, and (2) we can choose to replace a harmful mindlessness practice with a less harmful one. For example, I know a young man who chose to read science fiction novels instead of entertaining suicidal fantasies.

The Buddhist path is known as "the Middle Way," and mindlessness practices can serve as a kind of middle way. For example, a client I worked with chose to iron as a way to "get a break" from her depression. She would "zone out" in front of the television and iron dinner napkins that were already well pressed. She could not be described as being mindful, but she was able to relax a bit. Then, when she was ready, she could once again bring her mindfulness to her arising experience. This choice also allowed her to develop some *maitri*. By choosing to give herself a break she was cutting the habit of self-aggression, which underlied her depression, as well.

THE OUTCOME

Usually it is time to end the therapeutic relationship when clients are able to continue on their own. Some may choose to develop a formal meditation practice, but many do not. Still, they have learned something about how to cultivate mindfulness and *maitri*. As clients develop increasing mindfulness and *maitri,* they are able to see more clearly into the details of their own habitual patterns. They are able to bring mindfulness to intense states of mind and are able to tolerate the openness, uncertainty, and anxiety that accompanies letting go of habitual patterns.

I often see increases in unconditional confidence. That is, people develop confidence that is not based on their roles or specialized skills, which are impermanent, but rather that is derived from their recognition that they can fully experience all the moments of their lives, pleasant and unpleasant. This comes naturally from the repeated application of mindfulness. Mindfulness shows us that it *is* possible to experience it all.

Frequently an outcome of therapy is the uncovering of the desire to benefit others. Reconnecting with our natural compassion is an outgrowth of becoming more at home with ourselves. In this way *maitri* toward ourselves tends to extend outward to others.

The outcome might not be the same thing as the removal of symptoms, but it might very well be a change in the relationship the person has to those symptoms. As Buddhism teaches, it is not the presence of pain that is the biggest problem: It is our struggle against it that causes suffering.

A Clinical Example

I had the opportunity of late to work with a woman, Marcia, whose mother had recently died. Marcia came to see me because she was shocked by the overwhelming grief she was experiencing. It seemed out of proportion to her, given that her relationship with her mother had lacked warmth and genuine contact of any kind. In fact, as she told me her history it was clear that her mother had at least colluded in allowing Marcia's alcoholic father to terrorize and demean her. From him Marcia heard endless descriptions of her inadequacy. Some part of her never fully believed the stories of her basic badness, yet they left their mark. After her father's death, Marcia became the primary caregiver for her increasingly helpless mother. Marcia had no memories of affection, support, or even kindness from her mother. Yet she was weeping and grief-ridden. It made no sense to her.

Unlike some of the previous clinical examples in which the clients were severely challenged by extreme states of mind, Marcia is an intelligent woman who has been extremely successful in life. In the ordinary sense, she is eminently sane. She is happily married, has earned advanced degrees, and runs her own business. She has engaged in therapy before and has, at times in her life, engaged in mindfulness practices such as yoga. Despite her insight (which was profound) into the impact of her childhood on her later life, Marcia felt devastated, and the devastation was bewildering.

Our work together involved creating a mindfulness practice of reviewing both her mother's and her own life stories. We brought to this task all of the mindfulness of body, feelings, and mind that we could. We consciously chose to track not only Marcia's experience in the moment, but also my experience to the extent that it might reveal exchange.

Despite contemplative psychotherapy's emphasis on working in the present, sometimes the way to do this is by bringing present mindfulness and awareness to old information.

First, we told the story of Marcia's mother's life as it was seen from the point of view of Marcia's mother. Slowly we came to see the deep pain of this woman who had seen no options in her narrow world. As Marcia did this, she was able first to track anger and frustration toward her mother. This was not new. What came later was a sense of compassion. How utterly painful it must have been to feel so trapped and alone. Her withdrawal into alcohol and mindless needlepointing became more understandable. With understanding came tenderness. Sometimes both of us would feel wordless sorrow.

Then, we turned to Marcia's own experience. We worked with spontaneous imagery that arose as we talked. In one image, Marcia described a sense of still feeling her mother present, clinging to her back similar to a baby with claws. We focused always on Marcia's experiences in the present moment as she noticed the contents of her mind. How could she touch the feelings that accompanied the images? Marcia worked with mindfulness of body and breath to see that the painful memories, the oppressive imagery, and her responses to them were all happening in the moment. Our relationship with each other provided a container and a sense of connectedness that she had lacked growing up.

She was able to open to these feelings, to experience them fully. This contrasted with what was now a less helpful habit of analyzing them, which she had developed in response to her father's abusiveness. (It had been quite helpful then and reflected her brilliant sanity at the time.)

In addition to touching, we also worked with letting go. Marcia used the outbreath as one way to do this. Another way she came up with was to work directly with the images, especially one of her mother failing to leave this world and go into death. Marcia designed a ritual to accompany her mother across a "line" into the receiving hands of already-deceased relatives. The point here is not the details of the ritual, although they were important; the point is that Marcia brought her attention and openness to her present experience as she worked with the memories, the images, and her feelings. Out of that came a creative response: the ritual, which she performed at home.

Another outcome was Marcia saying, "It really was that bad, wasn't it?" Until now, she had known the story, but she had kept the pain at bay by intellectualizing it and keeping her distance from her childhood home. Her recognition of how bad things really were reflects the First and Second Noble Truths: seeing the truth of suffering and understanding that trying to escape it brings still more suffering. Marcia's path included mindfulness of body and also the technique of touch and go. In what was one of our last sessions, Marcia described what she first called "contentment." She later clarified it as "tenderness." She had also discovered that she no longer needed to be such an accomplished person. She could continue to do what she had passion for, but she no longer had to disprove the stories of being bad that she had heard from her abusive father. In these ways Marcia glimpsed the Third Noble Truth, the cessation of suffering, and she acquired some tools of mindfulness and *maitri* to help her continue on her path.

A Client's Own Description

A man who worked with a contemplative psychotherapist was kind enough to write the following description of his own experience of therapy and its outcomes. He had entered therapy because of acute anxiety and paralyzing feelings of depression.

> Not struggling against my fears and aversions was contrary to very deep impulses. But in therapy I was able to do so with [my therapist's] help. To actually stay with the immediacy of the moment's emotion while talking and thinking about life's terrors was transformative. The fear dissipated, my outlook about myself and my world softened, and instead of panic about the exterior situations in my life, I began to feel tender and sad—signs to me of true acceptance. The sadness was wholly different from my depressions. . . . In its essence, my therapy was an intensive tutorial in the practice of mindfulness—the technique of staying with the moment. With help I became much more aware of the workability of "now."

This man points to another important outcome of successful contemplative psychotherapy: the recognition that we are all workable just as we are. Workability implies that we are open to our experience, that we are willing to see it clearly, and that we regard ourselves with compassion. When we see that we are workable, we are on the path to uncovering our brilliant sanity.

REFERENCES

Chodron, P. (1994). *Start Where You Are: A Guide to Compassionate Living.* Boston: Shambhala.

Fortuna, J. (1987). Therapeutic Households. *The Journal of Contemplative Psychotherapy,* IV, 49-73.

Hanh, T. N. (1990). Buddhism and Psychotherapy: Planting Good Seeds. *The Journal of Contemplative Psychotherapy,* VII, 97-107.

Karthar, K. 1992. *Dharma Paths* (Trans. N. Burkhar and C. Radha). Ithaca, NY: Snow Lion.

Maitreya, A. and Asanga, A. (1985). *The Ultimate Mahayana Treatise on the Changeless Continuity of the True Nature: The Changeless Nature: Mahayana Uttara Tantra Sastra* (Trans. K. Holmes and K. Holmes). Scotland: Karma Drubgyud Darjay Ling (originally published 1979).

McLeod, K. (1989). Apples and Bricks? Some Differences Between Buddhism and Psychotherapy. *Journal of Contemplative Psychotherapy,* VI, 29-44.

Podvoll, E. (1983). The History of Sanity in Contemplative Psychotherapy. *Naropa Institute Journal of Psychology,* II, 11-32.

Podvoll, E. (1990). *The Seduction of Madness: Revolutionary Insights into the World of Psychosis and a Compassionate Approach to Recovery at Home.* New York: Harper and Row.

Reps, P. and Senzaki, N. (1957). *Zen Flesh, Zen Bones.* Boston: Tuttle Publishing.

Steven, J. (Trans.) (1981). *One Robe, One Bowl: The Zen Poetry of Ryoken,* Sixth Printing. First Edition 1977. New York: John Weatherhill, Inc.

Trungpa, C. (1987). *Cutting Through Spiritual Materialism.* Boston: Shambhala.

Trungpa, C. (1991). *The Heart of the Buddha.* Boston: Shambhala.

Watson, G., Batchelor, S., and Claxton, G. (Eds.) (1999). *The Psychology of Awakening: Buddhism, Science and Our Day-to-Day Lives.* London: Rider.

Wegela, K. K. (1988). Touch and Go in Clinical Practice: Some Implications of the View of Intrinsic Health for Psychotherapy. *The Journal of Contemplative Psychotherapy,* V, 3-23.

Wegela, K. K. (1996). *How to Be a Help Instead of a Nuisance: Practical Approaches for Giving Support, Service and Encouragement to Others.* Boston: Shambhala.

Wegela, K. K. and Joseph, A. (1992). Shock, Uncertainty, Conviction: Gateways Between Psychopathology and Intrinsic Health. *The Journal of Contemplative Psychotherapy,* VIII, 33-52.

CHRISTIANITY

You shall love the Lord [your] God with all [of your] heart, and with all [of your] soul, and with all [of your] strength, and with all [of your] mind; and your neighbor as [yourself].

Luke 10:27 (*The Holy Bible,* King James Version)

Christianity's golden rule asks us to love the Divine Presence with all of our consciousness, and to love humanity as we love ourselves. In this troubled world many of us do not know how to love ourselves. If we lack a sense of our own value, we lose the capacity to receive divine love within our hearts and bodies. Because of this "halfheartedness," we lose the connection to the foundation of love. Jesus' guidance is very direct. It describes a complete experience of love—psychological and spiritual.

The lives of the Christian mystics offer examples for dealing with life's complexities and also illuminate the way to mystical union. Jesus taught that heaven was within each one of us. How can the Christian client or student find this "heaven within" and experience the deepest healing possible? Dwight Judy's chapter encourages the reader to explore the use of contemplative prayer practices for the awakening of the power of Christ as healer within the psyche. Teachers, ministers, priests, and therapists can all use these examples to help their students and clients to heal.

In his chapter, Judy discusses psychospirituality from a Christian perspective and emphasizes the role of faith, prayer, and imagery in psychospiritual healing. The powerful healing focus of prayer should not be underestimated. In the emerging paradigm of integrative health, Larry Dossey and other researchers (1999) have demonstrated the healing results of prayer and its effects upon spiritual, psychological, and physical healing.

Drawing on practices of interior life that can be traced to the earliest application of Christianity, Judy shows how the practitioner can develop a pathway of a healing relationship with the interior Christ drawing on the wisdom of Scripture as well as present experience. This potentiality can facilitate the healing of emotional distress, help in the discernment of life direction, and also ease the dying process. Christian practice above all invites each individual into a direct healing relationship with this inner Christ, a relationship that brings healing love and presence to one's own experience of life.

Chapter 2

Rediscovering Christ, the Healer

Dwight H. Judy

meditation continued to be present with her for several hours that night. In her inner vision experience, Christ was with her. Christ calmed her anxiety as her memories unfolded again of the traumatic encounter in the hospital, and she watched inwardly as she began the birthing process. She relived her physical contractions. Christ comforted and sustained her and in her interior experience gave her the great gift she had longed for, to participate consciously in the birth of that child. Her physical and her emotional life were changed by this visitation of Christ, the Healer.

This experience occurred spontaneously only a few years ago. We are accustomed to thinking of such experiences as being locked away in the mystical writings of previous generations, rather than as a part of our spiritual resources for today. However, as will be discussed in this chapter, this type of experience is not uncommon in our time. Whether evoked through meditative prayer, through guided imagery experiences, or spontaneously, an interior visitation of Christ, the Healer, is a potentiality that is very much with us. We will search together to understand and apply this healing resource.

It is only in recent centuries that Western Christianity has lost connection with Christ as a "living," transpersonal healer. Yet as this experience illustrates, people in our time have begun again to experience healing encounters with Christ within their inner lives. The numerous healing stories of Jesus recorded in Scripture may now be looked upon in new light, based on current biblical scholarship. The recovery of methods of Christian prayer have also awakened a new experience for many people. In the early twentieth century, biblical scholarship was very skeptical of the veracity of the healing stories of Jesus. Today, a new image is emerging that gives credence to the historical Jesus as a person of great healing power (Borg, 1994).

In the first century of Christianity, it was common for early Christians to experience healings within their midst. Many of these experiences are recorded in Scripture. In this chapter we examine a way to understand the potentiality that Jesus carried in life a healing power, which was carried beyond his death within the capacity of collective human experience. How can Christ yet be an agent of healing? We shall seek to understand this potentiality. It will involve some excursion into the history of Christian prayer, as well as the present experiences of those undergoing such healings. Throughout this exploration, a theory of transpersonal psychotherapeutic practice will be described through which we might understand these experiences.

The link from earliest Christianity to the present time in understanding the presence of Christ as healer is through a newly discovered lineage of contemplative prayer practice. In the past twenty years, Christianity has recovered what it had almost lost in this century: an understanding of its own lineage of mysticism. This recovery includes the reclamation of descriptions of inner experience that appear in the very earliest centuries of Christianity during a very sophisticated period in the High Middle Ages, as well as during the period of the Reformation. When we trace these sources we find that often in Christian history it has been very common for prayer to be offered directed toward Christ in the interior imagination. This practice was particularly well attested during the sixteenth century in the writings of Ignatius of Loyola (Mottola, 1964) and Teresa of Avila (Kavanaugh and Rodriguez, 1976, 1980, 1985). These and other teachers of Christian mystical life offered understandings of the spiritual dynamics of prayer and the challenge of living one's life faithfully before God in all things. Their use of imagining Christ in prayer was so common that it obviously was the normal way to pray. Even so, throughout Christian history these methods of prayer have been more common among monastics than among laypersons. Their usage has suffered during periods when intellectualism has been in ascendancy within the church. Our current time period is unique both in seeking a balance between mystical and intellectual understandings as well as in bringing spiritual resources from the world's religious traditions into the experience of any earnest seeker. The recovery of prayer through imagination is the link to assist us to access Christ as a healing presence at the present time. The human psyche allows continuity from the historical person of Jesus Christ to this transhistorical experience in contemporary life.

REDISCOVERING MYSTICAL CHRISTIANITY

A dramatic shift has been taking place in the past thirty ye within Christian practice. The methods of contemplative pray gether with the rediscovery of the writings of the Christian throughout the ages, have brought forth a new depth ex prayer and interior knowing that had been absent for s ticularly within Western Christian life (Fox, 1980, 19 Thomas Merton (1915-1968) was a key catalyst in this ng rediscovery of mystical Christianity. Many others have follwed. Merton's book, *Contemplative Prayer* (1990), was one of the most important statements in the twentieth century for recovering Christian prayer. He reintroduced many of the Christian mystics and also interpreted the religions of the East to Christians in the Western world. Today, extensive training programs in various denominations focus on the renewal of prayer. The general term with which this renewal is being described is *spiritual formation*.

A very large lay movement under the leadership of Father Thomas Keating of Snowmass, Colorado, now teaches a simple meditative prayer technique called *centering prayer* (1991a,b, 1992; Pennington, 1980). In addition, the Ignatian retreat model continues to thrive in many locations. People in a variety of settings are being taught the practices of prayer and silence that lead to an awakening of the inner life. Bookstores carry a multitude of writings from Christian sources on both historical and contemporary applications of contemplative prayer (Bakken, 2000; Dossey, 1993; Fox, 1980, 1983, 1991, 1992; Flinders, 1993; French, 1952; Johnston, 1973; Kadloubovsky and Palmer, 1954; Kavanaugh and Rodriguez, 1976; Morello, 1991; Nouwen, 1974; Underhill, 1990).

Bonaventure (thirteenth century) noted that humanity has the capacity for three modes of perception: the eye of reason, the eye of the senses, and the eye of contemplation (Cousins, 1978). In the nineteenth and twentieth centuries, Western intellectual life focused much attention on the eye of reason and the eye of the senses. What Bonaventure meant by describing these as "eyes" is that they were innate capacities that needed to be cultivated to develop fully. Much of our schooling as children and adolescents is directed toward awakening the eye of reason more fully. The arts contribute to the awakening of the eye of the senses. The empirical method in science combines acute sensory perception with reason.

Through prayer we learn to open the eye of contemplation. Only through attention to the inner world will we learn how to navigate its waters, with their swirls of images, feelings, and motivations. That navigation of the inner life is precisely the task and challenge when we begin to open this eye of contemplation through regular prayer practice.

A notable figure in the recovery of Christian spiritual imagination has been Morton Kelsey. An Episcopal priest and a Jungian psychologist, Kelsey began the lonely task over twenty years ago of calling attention to the potential of inner life that lay dormant within Christianity. In *The Other Side of Silence* (1976), Kelsey made a fascinating assertion. He called the inner life the "psychoid" world. He wrote, the "key" to the psychoid world is imagination.

Kelsey was pointing out what Carl Jung had discovered as well: There lies within us a latent potentiality of subtle imagination process, very ready to cooperate with our inner drive for wholeness. Our dream life proceeds from this realm of the psyche, as well as that type of interior imagination that opens up in guided imagery experiences, or what Jung cultivated as "active imagination." Kelsey rediscovered that Christian tradition had known of a similar process for centuries.

In this Christian prayer practice, most fully described in *The Spiritual Exercises of St. Ignatius* (Mottola, 1964), it is taken for granted that we can enter into a state of prayer and communicate with Christ. A most effective way to do so is to utilize stories and images of Christ in Scripture. In the sixteenth century, Ignatius gave directions on building up the inner sensory experience to make it more vivid. Ignatius would have been quite at home with current practitioners of guided imagery as they have relearned this practice of developing the interior senses to make new discoveries from the treasury of the psyche regarding a particular problem or illness. This practice is also well attested in the writings of Teresa of Avila, who also lived in the sixteenth century. She frequently advocated visiting Christ in prayer and bringing the particular struggles or issues of the moment into that experience. She suggested that we should identify our mood, find a matching image of Christ from a Scripture story, and then pray with that Scripture image to help work through our struggles. In her most mature writing, "Interior Castle" (see Kavanaugh and Rodriguez, 1980), Teresa likened the soul to an interior castle with many rooms. She taught that the soul becomes more aware of itself through prayer and contemplation and described the innermost room of our being as the place where God dwells. Teresa taught that our discovery of this inner "guest," or Christ, would be the most important discovery of our lives; once we realize that God is dwelling within us, we are given both great personal authority and the understanding of seeking Divine guidance for all of our activities. When a client or person of prayer has been touched by this Presence, he or she will then know that there is an eternal purpose to one's life beyond any current depression, anxiety, or relational disturbance.

New resources are also emerging from present biblical scholarship that assist Christianity to understand its mystical roots more fully. Fascinating new material is beginning to surface from a new "quest for the historical Jesus." This task has challenged biblical scholars for well over a century. The first attempts to identify the historical Jesus were influenced by scholars of the nineteenth century who first began to recognize the difficulty of penetrating the biblical texts to the authentic record of Jesus. As biblical scholarship uncovered a variety of sources for various texts, and as the sequence of different texts in terms of their time of writing began to be questioned, much of our understanding of the Bible was thrown into confusion (Borg, 1994). Could we trust that the words of Jesus in our Bibles, those words highlighted in red, were actually the words of the historical man called Jesus? Furthermore, linguistic issues were considered more deeply; layers of translation lay between us in our time and a man who lived 2,000 years ago.

In this first search for the historical Jesus, there was much debate regarding the authenticity of Jesus as a healer. It became fashionable to declare that no such healings could have occurred—that they were an artifact of the ancient world and the way great people were described then. Healing stories were placed in the same category for some as stories of miraculous births—namely, in the category of a literary device used to describe extraordinary people. It seemed that we were receiving images of the historical man, Jesus, tainted by the cultural norms of the time. Essentially, it wrote off any aspect of the "miraculous" because those things "don't happen" in the present-day world, so they must not have happened in the ancient world either. Jesus, the healer, was relegated to a footnote of the "real" Jesus, a significant teacher and prophet whose life was distorted through the popular literary devices of those who wrote about him.

A new quest for the historical Jesus is currently under way in the material arising from the Jesus Seminar. The Jesus Seminar is an ongoing meeting of biblical scholars that focuses on comparing texts from Matthew, Mark, Luke, and the recently discovered Gospel of Thomas, one of the Dead Sea Scrolls. Marcus Borg (1994), one of the scholars of the Jesus Seminar, has been particularly vocal regarding his interpretation that the healing stories of Jesus are historically accurate portrayals of a great healer. Borg has also been influenced by holy men and women in the Hindu tradition. In other words, now, in our time, through intercultural understandings, the West is able to rewrite its own perception of what is possible for human beings to experience. A place for the miraculous is again being made in the West. Furthermore, Borg is clear that the scholarship itself now points to the authenticity of Jesus as a healer. Using the same criteria used for authenticating other material of Jesus' teaching, such as the Beatitudes, the Lord's Prayer, and many of the parables, it is necessary also to say that Jesus healed people.

CONTEMPORARY PRAYER EXPERIENCES

With this brief background, some healing prayer experiences will be explored, and then we will turn our attention again to seek to understand the process of prayer healing.

A man who has considerable experience with prayer was confronted with a very difficult process in his work life. In the midst of this situation, an opportunity came for him to be away, which offered longer periods for reflection than usual for him. As he spent time silently struggling with this issue, the image came to him of Jesus casting rocks out from his heart. After a period of time during which the rocks were cast away, the man was then filled with a sense of light and joy. The next day, although the problem continued to occupy some of his attention, he was also filled with a sense of joy, as well as relief from being less consumed by the problem.

A man suffered from a chronic headache, which troubled him daily. He was guided into a meditation from Scripture with Christ present. He had never before experienced this type of inner meditation with Christ. As he found himself before Christ, he asked earnestly to be healed. The relationship between the man and Christ was clarified in the inner experience as one of companionship and friendship. At the end of the meditation, he and Christ threw their arms around each other's shoulders and walked off laughing together. His headache symptoms disappeared for three days, a miracle for him at the time.

A couple, in the midst of trying to decide which avenues to pursue for adoption of a child, asked Christ for advice in prayer. They received guidance which helped them choose the route to take. Following this advice, the adoption was pursued successfully.

What is happening in these types of experiences? I have guided people into the imaginative representation of Christ now for almost twenty years in retreat settings (see Photo 2.1). It has universally surprised me that when approached in this way, persons receive advice that is generally wise counsel. They receive a different perspective on the problem or issue. They actually receive, in many cases, some physical release from symptoms. Usually, there is an element of surprise in the encounter with Christ and usually wisdom beyond what was expected is received. To seek an answer to the question of what is happening in these encounters, we need to look both to the inherent psychological functions of the person as well as the arena of spiritual encounter. However, we will find these explorations more fruitful if we first examine Jesus' healing presence in Scripture.

When we examine the biblical descriptions of Jesus as a healer, we witness a remarkable parallel to current thought in body-mind process. Often Jesus asks the person how the symptoms should be addressed—as a spiritual problem or as a physical problem—in essence, "Shall I tell you your sins are forgiven, or shall I heal your

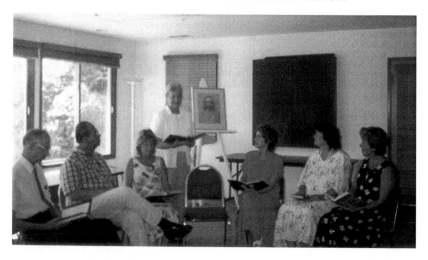

PHOTO 2.1. Christian study group. Courtesy of the Christward Ministry at Questhaven Retreat, Escondido, California.

physical infirmity?" For Jesus, it is clear that what we separate as spiritual and physical dimensions are one and the same process. If he heals spiritually or addresses the deep psychological conflict needing forgiveness, the physical healing in many cases will follow. We also see incidents of healing of mental disorders or casting out of demonic presences in Scripture. Frequently, a person asks for healing on his or her own behalf. In fact, frequently it seems to be the person's persistence that is rewarded. Some people ask for healing on behalf of others.

The story of the healing of the centurion's servant (Matthew 8:5-13) is perhaps the most important in terms of understanding the potentiality for present-day healing. A man comes and asks Jesus to heal his servant. Jesus answers that he will go to him, but the centurion replies that he need not, for he trusts that Jesus need "only say the word," and the man will be healed. Jesus thus engages in what we would today call, "remote healing." He does not need to be physically present to provide healing.

In present times, there is another theme of Christian experience that we must explore to draw contemporary applications: the reports of Jesus' appearances after his death. Did Jesus truly rise from the dead? Unmistakably, he "appeared." These appearances in some cases had a distinctly physical manifestation. In other cases, they seem more mystical in nature. In the records of Scripture, there is a great variety in these appearances, ranging from seemingly physical manifestations to more ephemeral experiences in which Jesus appears and then disappears after a message has been given. People are also instructed on spiritual matters within their dreams. Over the past twenty years, I have personally listened to many people describe their encounters with Christ. Even in our time some have reported a physical presence, for example, Christ being present in the room and then leaving in some distinctive manner. More frequently, individuals report an inner visionary experience. Is the Christ appearing now, whether fully physically present or present in inner vision, the same Christ that appeared to his faithful following his death?

In my early thirties, I encountered a woman in the midst of such a mystical manifestation. It was early on Easter morning. I was pastor of the woman, also in her thirties, who lay dying in the hospital of a congenital heart problem. I had witnessed her decline during the previous year. It had only been a few Sundays earlier that I began to recognize how very fragile she had become. It was the custom in the congregation for laypersons to walk to the pulpit to read the Scripture lesson. That Sunday, this young woman read. As she walked with feeble and halting steps to the pulpit, I finally realized that she was losing her battle to live. That Easter morning, as I walked into the hospital room, she was very weak but radiant. As she greeted me, she said, "You are Christ today."

I, of course, recognized that she was not talking about me personally, but that the radiance within the room that I, too, was experiencing, was indeed "Christ" to her. For her, Christ had come to usher her through the gateway of death, which came a few days later. This experience profoundly changed my perspective on the possibility for mystical experiences to arise within persons in our time. It suggested to me that these experiences of divine light, radiant presence, or "essential" energy might bring profound power with them to change our emotional, physical, and spiritual realities. In other words, this experience awakened me to the potentiality of mystical healing. I needed to find my own understanding of how to make sense of this type of phenomenon in our time.

These profound issues are very difficult to understand. Are we dealing with a Christ presence which is such a part of the essential human collective experience that there is a completely psychological explanation? Does the answer somehow lie within our understanding of a collective unconscious for all of humanity as a repository of all human experience? Is Christ a "living" entity within this arena who continues to manifest to those earnestly petitioning for help, or is Christ a manifestation of our more personal minds built up from our understanding of various teachings we have encountered throughout our lives?

One Buddhist meditation teacher shared that, in her experience, Christ always appeared in the meditation of Westerners at the point in which they were working deeply to access the spirit of compassion in their Buddhist practice. My point is to suggest that one explanation for Christ's continuing appearance may be the ontological explanation suggested by the Gospel of John. In this great metaphysical writing, John writes that the creative energy through which all things were created was manifest in the man, Jesus, and thus "Christ" is eternal, preceding Jesus' historical life, and present now and in all futures. According to John's understanding this universal Divine Presence is the core of an ongoing creative life force which enlivens every living thing.

> When all things began, the Word already was. The Word dwelt with God, and what God was, the Word was. The Word, then, was with God at the beginning, and through him all things came to be; no single thing was created without him. All that came to be was alive with his life, and that life was the light of [humankind]. The light shines on in the dark, and the darkness has never mastered it. (John 1:1-5, *New English Bible* [NEB])

In this description of creation, we may say the "light" of Christ, or the regenerating power of creative renewal, is inherently present in every created being. Thus, when we experience an outpouring of the divine creative energy, we are simply touching that which is present in potentiality at every moment of creation. When the divine life energy manifests in our own visionary life as Christ, Jesus is bringing the potentiality for re-creation, which is inherently present in us through our own biological life process. What enables us to be alive? What allows our cells to regenerate? For the person steeped in mystical Christianity, we may say that Christ brings this potentiality present fully in the moment in which we experience this Divine Presence. For some people, in some circumstances, Christ will be present to the external senses. For some, Christ will be present in an inner vision. For others, there will be only a figure of light that they will identify as Christ. It is very helpful that the Gospel of John itself speaks of this Presence as "light," because in many cases the manifestation of "light" or "Presence" is what is given, rather than a description of a particular figure.

My experience is that ordinarily these encounters are nonpathological in nature. They can bring healing, insight, and clarity. They may occur without schizoid or delusional manifestations. Instead, they represent an answer to a deeply held need, usually bringing an extraordinary clarity and sense of well-being with them. Some persons seem particularly gifted in prayer healing and may be the agent for bringing this powerful regenerative energy directly to the person in need. The contemporary church has also been in the process of reclaiming the ritual of a liturgy for healing. Such times of worship may bring the healing sense of Divine Presence very fully alive.

There are occasions in which this Christ Presence seems to be co-opted into a psychotic episode. I once witnessed an incident in which a man was unable to receive sedation following surgery due to an acute asthmatic condition. As his sleep deprivation continued over several days due to severe pain, he first seemed comforted by a Christ Presence with him. Over the course of the next few days, however, his experience became paranoid in nature. What he espoused to be Christ communicating to him did not relate to the Christ as healing presence that I have witnessed in the many healthy encounters I have observed through the years. This Jesus also began to deviate markedly from the compassionate Jesus reported in Scripture—always a test for Christian discernment. The individual was hospitalized briefly in a mental institution to help his mental recovery after he was able to be released from the hospital for his physical condition. His paranoid ideation did not return after he was able to receive adequate rest.

Thus there may be a limit to the power of the Christ "light" as perceived by the individual. Major psychotic episodes may limit the effectiveness of Christ to bring healing and comfort. However, for the person with reasonably healthy psychological functioning, Christ may appear in any of the manifestations I have been describing with a sense of wisdom, guidance, and well-being.

PRAYER HEALING WITH SCRIPTURE STORIES

The most universal method of evoking Christ, the healer, is through those stories in Scripture in which it is reported that Jesus performed healings. Some of those include: the healing of Peter's mother-in-law (Matthew 8:14-15; Mark 1:29-31), the healing of the hemorrhaging woman (Matthew 9:20-22; Mark 5:25-34; Luke 8:43-48), the healing of the man lame for thirty-eight years (John 5:1-16), and the release from mental torment to the man possessed by Legion (Mark 5:1-20).

The method is to utilize the story to build the inner experience of the person who is entering into prayer. In doing so, Ignatius of Loyola, in his *Spiritual Exercises* (Mottola, 1964), encourages us to utilize all of the internal senses—to build the inner story by inviting our inner imagination to build up sounds, smells, physical sensations, and pictures. In entering into this process, it is useful to note that people have different inner responses, that some people will be highly visual while others will receive their information more through auditory or kinesthetic modes. Thus, the advice to build all of the senses is quite sound, because through doing so everyone will find a dominant inner sense that will manifest (Achterberg, 1985; Achterberg, Dossey, and Kolkmeier, 1994).

It is also useful to recognize that as the figure of Jesus enters the scene, he is sometimes only a figure of light, sometimes quite faint, and sometimes very graphically human in his characteristics.

As we enter the story, we allow the scene to give us a root metaphor with which we can bring forth our current life issue. Thus, the paralysis of the man lame for thirty-eight years will for some reflect a physical problem with which they are struggling. For others it may be an emotional process. For some it may be a very particular relational problem that is currently troubling them. For others it might be a recurrent vocational struggle. The genius of the method begins to manifest at this point. By taking the element of suffering within the story as root metaphor, we are able to bring our current life issues into the scene. Then, when Christ encounters us, we listen, we pray, we ask advice, and we experience the possibility of receiving new insight and clarity on the issue.

For some, the Divine Presence of Christ will manifest an energy that is very strong. It may take them into a new relationship with their bodies. It may seem to flood them with light. For others it will be a very subtle experience. The insights may come in simple ways, such as noticing what age they are when they begin to enter the story or where they are. In other words, we have entered that arena of the psyche in which information may be given through subtle cues, similar to dream material. It may require analysis—similar to dream analysis following prayer to understand its full impact.

FREE-FORM PRAYER HEALING

Another way to apply these processes is to use a prayer healing intention without using a setting from a Scripture story. In many cases, when entering into deep life material, one of the helping figures that may manifest spontaneously is Christ. When that happens, we are usually in the arena of Christ, the Healer, manifesting. At that point, the situation becomes a practice of co-therapy, in which Christ becomes the key therapeutic agent. As external counselor, I shift my role to be less directing and more inviting to perceive what it may be that Christ is seeking to unfold in the inner world of the individual.

A significant way to enter this world is to invite the prayer petitioner to identify the key life issue or physical symptom or problem needing attention. Then we enter into a spirit of meditation or prayer through some simple relaxation process—often taking a few full breaths is enough. Next, the petitioner is invited to allow an image, symbol, or word to arise that expresses this problem area. With a little prompting, particularly in avoiding self-censure, usually a root image will come quickly. At this point it is usually helpful to ask if the image can give information itself or if it needs a helper to express itself. In many cases, Christ will be brought forth spontaneously as the helper. Another wisdom figure can appear as the manifestation of the healing potentiality. In some cases, Christ will be invited in to assist in the healing process while a story evolves from the symbolic representation of the problem. With gentle probing, a childhood memory may surface. The symbol may hold the story fully within itself and be the theme needed to work out the process.

A particularly valuable process to use in the healing of childhood memory is to invite the "inner light" to be present with the child within the memory of a traumatic event. The manifestation may be Christ or a feminine Divine Presence or other inner wisdom figure with which the person is already familiar. In being thus present, the memory is often shifted so that the inner child is able to better handle the situation. It can also be very helpful to bring the image of the person as an adult into the childhood scene.

This type of prayer healing was utilized by Agnes Sanford (1984, 1990) early in the twentieth century. She was widely recognized as a Christian prayer healer with much integrity. Her influence was profound enough that many of her writings are still available, although she has been deceased for some time. This type of prayer experience is currently described in many exercises in the writings of Flora Slosson Wuellner (1987, 1992), who has particularly focused on interfacing prayer with the body and with emotional issues.

A way to enter into imagery prayer healing is to work with a particular Scripture text, such as the following:

> That day, in the evening, he said to them, "Let us cross over to the other side of the lake." So they left the crowd and took him with them in the boat where he had been sitting; and there were other boats accompanying him. A heavy squall came on and the waves broke over the boat until it was all but swamped. Now he was in the stern asleep on a cushion; they roused him and said, "Master, we are sinking! Do you not care?" He awoke, rebuked the wind, and said to the sea, "Hush! Be still!" The wind dropped and there was dead calm. He said to them, "Why are you such cowards? Have you no faith even now?" They were awestruck and said to one another, "Who can this be? Even the wind and the sea obey him." (Mark 4:35-41 NEB)

> Begin by imagining the scene of the boat by the shore. Take some time to fill in the details. The more of the inner senses you access, the more vivid your experience will be. Do not be discouraged if you do not have strong visual images. Some people seem to have vivid imagery; others do not seem to have vivid imagery, yet even so, by working with this method, they receive intriguing insights.
>
> As you imagine the scene by the shore, ask yourself to give the colors of the sky near dusk. Listen for the sound of the water on the shore line. Is the beach sandy or rocky? What is the temperature? Let your imagination give you your own picture of these circumstances. . . . Notice the two small boats described in the story ready to receive passengers. . . . Then, notice the people approaching the boats. Let your imagination give you your own picture of Jesus as he might have looked when he lived. See the others travelling with him. Let them embark on the boats in your imagination. . . . Notice that you now enter the story also

and find yourself a place on the boat where Jesus is riding. As the boats cast off, let the sky darken. Night sets in. . . . After a while, you and the others on the boat make beds for the night on the deck. Jesus finds a place and is asleep at the rear of the boat. You fall asleep. . . . You are awakened by violent tossing of the boat and by the water of the waves crashing onto the boat. You experience your terror and the terror of others and you wonder if you will survive. (Now, bring your own current life worries and anxieties into the story with you. What fears are you dealing with? Let yourself experience your fears and name them. Let your current life issues now enter into a dialogue with the images of the story.) You and others notice that Jesus is asleep in the rear of the boat, unaffected by the storm. Someone yells for him to wake up. Notice that he then gets up and says to the storm: "Hush! Be still!"

Here I leave my guidance for you to take your own prayer forward. Hear Jesus' words in the story as your inner meditation phrase: "Hush! Be still!" Hear him saying those words to your current fears and anxieties. This is a powerful method to cultivate the strength of the inner Christ. Can you let your inner Christ arise up to greater power than your anxieties and fears? "Hush! Be still!" Can you let yourself receive insights and creative solutions to those problems that are creating the anxieties and fears? (Judy, 1996, pp. 101-102)

Similar guided imagery experiences with Scripture are available in Morton Kelsey's *The Other Side of Silence* (1976) and in Carolyn Stahl Bohler's book, *Opening to God* (1996). People who find this kind of meditation useful sometimes like to make an audiotape of such a guided meditation and then use it to help them into the experience.

AN EXPERIENCE OF PRAYER HEALING

I have been describing methods for opening to the inner Christ of healing in particular times of prayer. I will now describe more fully the experience of the man who had the prayer experience of Christ casting rocks out from his heart. It will illustrate more completely the array of imagery that may emerge over time. Our experience is rarely limited to one moment of personal understanding and healing; more ordinarily, when we are dealing with complex issues, we can witness an unfolding over time, which will draw on a wide spectrum of inner psychological, physical, and spiritual themes.

The spontaneous meditation of Christ casting out rocks really began with a history about two years earlier. The man had been in the most grueling experience of his life's work, being under attack in a very challenging way by another person within his work life. During that time, he came to realize that he could not address the situation effectively through personal communication. There was also a profound array of multigenerational issues at work. A large institution was involved and many persons were focusing intense energy toward it at the time. During this intensely stressful time, the man had prayed, asking for some peace concerning this issue. An image came in his dreams of a skeletal hand gripping his heart. At that point he realized how very treacherous this situation had become. In many encounters, there would be intense exchanges of anger, or in meetings distorted information relating to his performance would be presented. An image of Christ victorious over evil was a frequent companion to him during this time. In light of the skeletal hand image, he also began to notice feeling tightness around his heart. He asked a small circle of people to pray for the situation, as it seemed impossible to address through normal means.

A more humorous image also appeared. He had a dream image of a scorpion. On a morning jog, the man realized this scorpion was representative of his own capacity for anger and attack, which he hated to use but could employ when necessary. As he jogged along, the scorpion image found its way to his side on a leash. It could—in his imagination—grow as large as a big dog, or be smaller. This image proved very helpful later in the week, in yet another meeting, in which he realized he would very likely be under attack. During the meeting, he visualized his scorpion on its leash by his side. He could use this form of self-protection if needed, but he would do so only if things became terribly challenging. Things progressed well in the meeting without him needing to call upon the scorpion. Yet this image continued to assist him when needed.

At a conference after the most intense period of this encounter, he was guided to meditate on his heart in a visualization exercise in which people were asked to relate to a part of the body that seemed to need attention. There appeared an image of small green plants. At first this seemed like a positive image. However, he wondered what soil the plants might be growing in. He had begun to have general feelings of sluggishness and continued from time to time to be concerned about his heart. He wondered if the image of the soil in his heart might be an indication of increasing arterial plaque.

A year later the meditation came spontaneously of Christ casting rocks out of his heart. Soon after this image appeared, he had an annual physical and discovered that his cholesterol had, indeed, climbed up from the low 200 range to high 200s. His physician cautioned him on the danger of this, with the admonition to see what he could do with diet in the next three months, before he would recommend medication to reduce cholesterol levels.

Over the next few months, the man strenuously reduced fat intake, significantly increased dietary fiber, and very frequently used the meditation of Christ casting rocks out of his heart. His cholesterol responded with a dramatic drop, which he maintained in bloodwork one year later. It was interesting to the man, because although his weight had increased a bit from the low weight he achieved after the first three months of dieting, he did not feel the same sluggishness.

Recently the image of Christ has returned to this man, this time casting stones from his mind! He has interpreted this to mean that it is time to observe and change many basic thought patterns. In fact, the patterns of external challenge to him have manifested in a new working environment. All of these inner images assist him in his commitment not to reenter the climate of anger and attack that he experienced in the previous situation.

A TRANSPERSONAL MODEL OF CHRISTIAN PRAYER HEALING

Figure 2.1 is adapted from Ken Wilber's book *The Atman Project* (1980), one of the most thorough attempts at a lifelong psychological and spiritual developmental model. In the diagram the life journey is marked from birth and early childhood through the development of our mature ego into mature adulthood and finally death. We see that potential exists within us for accessing what is here called "symbolic" awareness, which links to the quality of imagination that we experience in early childhood and can return in our interior prayer of imagination, dreams, and visualization process in mature adulthood.

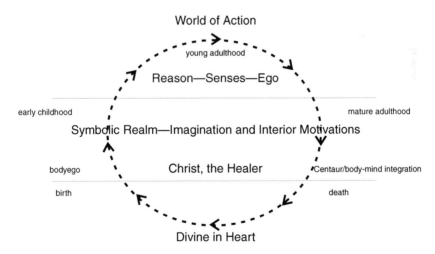

FIGURE 2.1. Adapted from Ken Wilber, *The Atman Project: A Transpersonal View of Human Evolution.* Wheaton, IL: Theosophical Publishing House, Quest. Reprinted by permission.

It is in this arena that Christ, the Healer, may appear to guide the inner process of understanding and integrating memory with emerging hope and physical awareness.

With respect to aspects of inner healing that have physical correlates, it is significant to note that Wilber postulates that our earliest "ego" identification of ourselves separately from our environment comes through our emerging identification with physiological process, which he terms the emergence of the "bodyego." This is a very primitive development within us, taking place around eighteen months to two years of age. It correlates in mature adulthood with the reconnection of mind and body in such a way that we can receive directly into our awareness physiological signals for health or disease. Wilber calls this body-mind integration by the name "Centaur," drawing on the mythological half-horse, half-human figure. We are able to be in tune with our physiological needs. The language of physical symptoms is often symbolic in nature. This particular arena of the psyche is opened through the types of meditation with imagination in Scripture stories that have been described (for more complete description, see Judy, 2000).

With the centuries of devotion to Christ that are embedded deeply within the collective human experience, it should not surprise us that this Christ figure would be imbued with the same healing power and wisdom as illustrated in the Scripture encounters with a living man called Jesus. Guidance is often given, with insight and clarity beyond our understanding or even beyond our power to ask for help.

MARY, THE SAINTS, AND OTHER WISDOM FIGURES

Within Roman Catholic tradition, there is often a similarly developed and highly powerful prayer to Mary for such healing and divine grace. This tradition is absent to a large degree in the Protestant world. It has been fascinating to me, as I have shared meditation experiences with so many people within Christian churches over the past twenty years, to discover how frequently Mary or another aspect of the Divine Mother or Divine Feminine Power has manifested spontaneously within people's experience in the present time. Although not fully acknowledged throughout mainstream Christianity, this emergence of the mystical Feminine Power is a very significant factor in our time. Often the inner healing process involves a profound encounter with an individual's understanding of the nature of God. We are heirs to a period of history, particularly in Western Christianity, in which this form has been almost exclusively masculine. Often it is essential to the deepest organization of the psyche to receive in a healthy way an inner understanding or vision of the Divine Feminine. This must frequently precede an integration with the Divine Masculine.

One of the most dramatic of these encounters with Mary occurs in the writings of Teresa of Avila.

> I saw our Lady at my right side and my father St. Joseph at the left, for they were putting that robe on me. I was given to understand that I was now cleansed of my sins. After being clothed and while experiencing the most marvelous delight and glory, it seemed to me then that our Lady took me by the hands. She told me I made her very happy in serving the glorious St. Joseph, that I would believe that what I was striving for in regard to the monastery would be accomplished, that the Lord and those two would be greatly served in it, that I shouldn't fear there would ever be any failure in this matter even though the obedience which was to be given was not to my liking, because they would watch over us, and that her Son had already promised us He would be with us, that as a sign that this was true she was giving me a jewel. . . . As for what the Queen of Angels said concerning obedience, it pertained to the fact that it distressed me not to give obedience to the order, but the Lord had told me it wasn't suitable to give it to my superiors. He gave me the reasons why it would in no way be fitting that I do so. But He told me I should petition Rome in a certain way, which He also indicated to me, and that He would take care that we get our request. And so it came about, for the petition was made the way the Lord told me and it was granted easily, whereas we had been unable to obtain it. (Kavanaugh and Rodriguez, 1980, pp. 226-227)

In this vision, Mary gives direction and protection for Teresa's life's work of creating small houses of prayer for women. The vision in prayer is unusual in the completeness it offers. Teresa has a sense of being forgiven of her sins and held in Divine Presence, but also given clarity about decisions she was trying to make in reference to the convents she was seeking to establish (Judy, 1996).

This type of prayer is "healing" to her sense of life purpose. It demonstrates, similar to the contemporary man's experience of Christ's direct encounter with the casting out of rocks from his heart and head, what can happen when people have developed a prayerful understanding of life. The prayer experiences can come spontaneously. We begin to be deeply connected to the highest wisdom, at the interface between human life and Divine Presence.

One of the most tragic elements in current Christian practice is a misunderstanding of the variety of ways both in Scripture and tradition that the Divine has manifested for healing in persons' life experience. When I use the image of "Christ, the healer," I truly mean Divine light, energy, and creative presence that may manifest in masculine, feminine, or nongender forms.

HEALING OF THE GENERATIONS— A NEW PERSPECTIVE ON PURGATORY

In the medieval Christian world, there were three realms of human existence—Hades, Purgatory, and Paradise—that might be our destination in death. They certainly were a way of describing the challenges of our human life in earthly existence. In Dante's *Divine Comedy* (1949, 1955, 1962), they were given marvelous form. Even the upper realms of Hades were a pleasant enough place. The only missing link for the dead in those realms, keeping them from Paradise, was the incapacity to envision life as an ecstatically joyous experience, the fullness of life that Dante perceived was given in Christ.

In Purgatory, persons worked through the deadly attitudes or "sins" that keep us so preoccupied and self-centered—attitudes such as hatred, greed, envy, pride, gluttony, lust, and sloth. Are those "lost souls" of our past still haunting us, still longing to be freed? As I work with people healing from childhood abuse, it frequently surfaces that this issue must be redeemed not only for the individual but also for their parental abuser or grandparents. We dwell in a vast web of life. It frequently occurs to me that we do not have a framework of such prayer for the dead in our time, as was the case in the medieval world.

There, with the concept of Purgatory, it was intended that we would continue to pray for the healing of those who had departed our world of time and space. My hope would be that in recovering the Christian practice of prayer healing we might look beyond the current generation to realize that in the sustained efforts many people must endure in their quest for personal healing, we are also reclaiming the ancient Christian practice of praying for the dead as we work through multigenerational patterns of abuse.

As persons worked through these challenges in Purgatory, they were not alone. Spiritual practices adapted to each problem were available, and angels assisted. For example, the angel of chastity watched over the healing of lust. The angel of generosity assisted the healing of envy. The angel of peace assists with the problem of anger. In our contemporary world, our therapist or spiritual director often serves this healing function, bringing insight and holding the prospect of healing before us, when we cannot yet perceive the whole dynamic of our struggle to envision a solution. Our strengths will be pointed out when we cannot perceive them. At some point, when successful, the bond of trust will be strong enough that we will reveal, perhaps for the first time even to ourselves, the trauma beneath our disease. In each of the realms—Hades, Purgatory, Paradise—Dante had a guide. We, too, will need guides when developing our access to these domains of depth that reveal themselves to us.

A number of years ago, traveling in Vera Cruz, Mexico, I entered a small cathedral. There I understood the inadequacies of current Western Christianity for so many. Upon the wall was a huge mural. It depicted people with all kinds of sufferings and needs reaching up from our earthly realm. Their hands were met by the hands of the saints and other departed souls who helped them mediate their human struggles to the direct Presence of Christ and the Holy Mother. That realm of intermediaries is often missing in our common vocabulary. We are recovering it in our experience with persons who hover near death. We may be recovering it in an understanding of our own inner helpers who can assist in a variety of forms. We may be blessed with the direct perception of God.

We are rediscovering the possibility of intermediaries of health when we entrust ourselves to a psychotherapist or spiritual director. The tradition of Christian spiritual direction through the centuries has encouraged our reaching out for such intermediary helpers.

INTERCESSORY PRAYER
AND THE LITURGY OF HEALING

One of the most enduring practices of Christian life has been the assumption that we would pray for one another when in distress. This practice is now being given authentication through the efforts of Larry Dossey (1993) and others who study the effects of prayer in times of disease. Emerging is a fascinating correlation of scientific data that supports prayer practice. This is "distance prayer." It is perhaps in the same arena of the functioning of the universe as Jesus' healing of the centurion's servant at a distance.

People often report in times of crisis—such as death or critical illness—that they have felt the support of the prayers of others. The benevolence of the universe has uplifted them. Although they cannot understand the nature of the universe that leads to such crisis, once within it they may feel the healing power of compassion surrounding them. They often attribute this experience to the prayers of others.

In many studies, the research is significant enough that Dossey suggests that for physicians not to recommend prayer along with other medical interventions is to practice inadequate medicine.

Such prayer is a mainstay for most Christians. In the worship life of the church, people are encouraged to pray for one another in times of crisis, illness, bereavement, and personal struggle. The church also prays over the hurts, struggles, and pains of the world. It is one of the few places in American culture where we can count on having the many needs of the world held up for prayer.

One way to pray that is quite accessible to many people is called centering prayer. In this prayer form, we open ourselves to the sense of Divine Presence, perceived as "love." Often we can feel this experience in the heart region. Then, in the prayer we offer this spirit of "love" to our thoughts as they flow through. We can anchor our minds with a simple work of phrase, such as "God," "love," "peace," and/or "Christ." When we use this as a form of intercessory prayer, we hold the person in need before this loving energy. It can also be profound for the individual offering prayer. Research increasingly supports the efficacy of this prayer as a contribution to the healing of others.

Many churches are reclaiming the early Christian practices of anointing with oil, laying on of hands, and offering prayers for healing and blessing. Often a very powerful sense of the Divine Presence occurs when groups of people open themselves to God in this way.

PRAYER IN A MYSTICAL COSMOS

Entering the new millennium, we are at a threshold, looking at potentialities for the integrative practice of spirituality and psychology. During the past thirty years, the West has been recovering a language of the soul, which had become virtually lost. The advances in transpersonal psychological theory of lifelong growth are combining with alternative therapeutic health practices, such as the studies on intercessory prayer, for the first time in modern history. Parallel to these developments, Western Christianity has itself reclaimed its living lineage of contemplative prayer practice. Very little work has yet been done in the integration of these two domains. Our understanding of the nature of our own cosmos is also emerging with fascinating constructs, which allows for the mysteries of inner awareness and healing that have been described.

In the therapeutic practice now occurring in so many psychotherapeutic offices, images of Christ, Mary, or other mystical Divine Presences may well emerge spontaneously. I trust that this chapter has given a small glimpse into the emerging field of Christian spiritual formation in which many resources for inner awareness, growth, healing, and historic methods of Christian prayer are now becoming available.

May our time be one of healing within our individual and collective areas of suffering that we might realize the ecstatic life envisioned by the Christian mystics throughout the centuries.

REFERENCES

Achterberg, J. (1985). *Imagery in Healing: Shaminism and Modern Medicine.* Boston: Shambhala.

Achterberg, J., Dossey, B., and Kolkmeier, L. (1994). *Rituals of Healing: Using Imagery for Health and Wellness.* New York: Bantam.

Bakken, Kenneth L. (2000). *The Journey into God: Healing and Christian Faith.* Minneapolis: Augsburg.

Bohler, Carolyn Stahl (1996). *Opening to God: Guided Imagery Meditation on Scripture.* Nashville: Upper Rom Books.

Borg, M. (1994). *Meeting Jesus Again for the First Time.* San Francisco: HarperSanFrancisco.

Cousins, E. (1978). *Bonaventure: The Soul's Journey into God, the Tree of Life, the Life of St. Francis* (Trans.). New York: Paulist Press.

Dante Alighieri (1949*). The Comedy of Dante Alighieri, the Florentine, Cantica I, Hell (Il Inferno)* (Trans. D. L. Sayers). New York: Penguin.

Dante Alighieri (1955). *The Comedy of Dante Alighieri, the Florentine, Cantica II, Purgatory (Il Purgatorio)* (Trans. D. L. Sayers). New York: Penguin.

Dante Alighieri (1962). *The Comedy of Dante Alighieri, the Florentine, Cantica III, Paradise (Il Paradiso)* (Trans. D. L. Sayers). New York: Penguin.

Dossey, L. (1993). *Healing Words: The Power of Prayer in the Practice of Medicine.* San Francisco: HarperSanFrancisco.

Dossey, L. (1999). *Beyond Mind-Body to a New Era of Healing.* San Francisco: HarperSanFrancisco.

Flinders, C. L. (1993). *Enduring Grace: Living Portraits of Seven Women Mystics.* San Francisco: HarperSanFrancisco.

Fox, M. (1980). *Breakthrough: Meister Eckhart's Creation Spirituality in New Translation.* Garden City, NY: Doubleday.

Fox, M. (1983). *Original Blessing: A Primer in Creation Spirituality.* Santa Fe: Bear and Co.

Fox, M. (1991). *The Coming of the Cosmic Christ.* San Francisco: HarperSanFrancisco.

Fox, M. (1992). *Sheer Joy: Conversations with Thomas Aquinas on Creation Spirituality.* San Francisco: HarperSanFrancisco.

French, R. M. (Trans.) (1952). *The Way of a Pilgrim and the Pilgrim Continues His Way,* Second Edition. Minneapolis: Seabury Press.

The Holy Bible, King James Version (n.d.). London: Cambridge University Press.

Johnston, W. (Ed.) (1973). *The Cloud of Unknowing and the Book of Privy Counseling.* Garden City, NY: Doubleday.

Judy, D. (1996). *Embracing God: Praying with Teresa of Avila.* Nashville: Abingdon.

Judy, D. (2000). *Christian Meditation and Inner Healing.* Akron, OH: OLS Publications.

Judy, D. (2003). *Quest for the Mystical Christ: Awakening the Heart of Faith.* Akron, OH: OSL Publications.

Kadloubovsky, E. and Palmer, G.E.H. (Eds. and Trans.) (1954). *Early Fathers from the Philokalia.* London and Boston: Faber.

Kavanaugh, K. and Rodriguez, O. (1976). *The Collected Works of St. Teresa of Avila,* Volume 1 (Trans.). Washington, DC: ICS Publications.

Kavanaugh, K. and Rodriguez, O. (1980). *The Collected Works of St. Teresa of Avila,* Volume 2. Washington, DC: ICS Publications.

Kavanaugh, K. and Rodriguez, O. (1985). *The Collected Works of St. Teresa of Avila,* Volume 3. Washington, DC: ICS Publications.

Keating, T. (1991a). *The Mystery of Christ: The Liturgy As Spiritual Experience.* Rockport, MA, and Shaftesbury, Dorset, UK: Element.

Keating, T. (1991b). *Reawakenings.* New York: Crossroad.

Keating, T. (1992). *Invitation to Love: The Way of Christian Contemplation.* Rockport, MA, and Shaftesbury, Dorset, UK: Element.

Kelsey, M. T. (1976). *The Other Side of Silence: A Guide to Christian Meditation.* New York: Paulist.

Kelsey, M. T. (1983). *Companions on the Inner Way: The Art of Spiritual Guidance.* New York: Crossroad.

Merton, T. (1960). *The Wisdom of the Desert.* New York: New Directions.

Merton, T. (1990). *Contemplative Prayer.* New York: Doubleday, Image.

Morello, A. (1991). Lectio Divina and the Practice of Teresian Prayer. *Spiritual Life, 37*(2): 84-100.

Mottola, A. (Trans.) (1964). *The Spiritual Exercises of St. Ignatius.* Garden City, NY: Doubleday, Image.

The New English Bible (1971). New York: Cambridge University Press.

Nouwen, H. J. M. (1974). *Out of Solitude: Three Meditations on the Christian Life.* Notre Dame, IN: Ave Maria Press.

Pennington, M. B. (1980). *Centering Prayer: Renewing an Ancient Christian Prayer Form.* Garden City, NY: Doubleday.

Sanford, A. (1984). *Healing Gifts of the Spirit.* San Francisco: HarperSanFrancisco.

Sanford, A. (1990). *The Healing Light.* New York: Ballantine.

Underhill, E. (1990). *Mysticism: A Study in the Nature and Development of Man's Spiritual Consciousness.* New York: Doubleday.

Wilber, K. (1980). *The Atman Project: A Transpersonal View of Human Evolution.* Wheaton, IL: Theosophical Publishing House, Quest.

Wuellner, F.S. (1987). *Prayer and Our Bodies.* Nashville: Abingdon.

Wuellner, F. S. (1992). *Heart of Healing, Heart of Light: Encountering God, Who Shares and Heals Our Pain.* Nashville: Upper Room.

GODDESS SPIRITUALITY

You walk upon my paths and acknowledge my beauty
But you do not know my power—
The power that can push forth mountain peaks
and open valleys for oceans to fill.

Gaia, our Mother Earth, seemed to be speaking through me as I recorded Her message. The words flowed without thought. I paused to await the next phrase and the Earth began to tremble beneath me. She was manifesting Her power, and I could feel it shaking the Earth.

This experience occurred a few months after the 1989 Oakland, California, earthquake. At the time I was living in a college dormitory in Oakland and was completing a homework assignment for a course in creative writing. We had been given the assignment of writing from the perspective of a plant, a piece of wood, or some other manifestation of nature. I made the decision to write as though I was the Earth Herself. The next morning I went for my sunrise walk in a redwood forest, returned to the dorm, and prepared to learn from the archetypal Goddess. In meditation I allowed the words to flow through me. They spoke of beauty, power, and metaphorically affirmed female sexuality. The earthquake synchronistically validated Her declaration.

If we examine the entirety of the world's female population, how many women would we find affirming this inherent spiritual and earthy power? This knowledge has the power to help women with limited identities heal. Because of the dominating influence of patriarchal religions, the majority of the Earth's female population has little, if any, awareness of the Goddess tradition. For this reason, feminist psychology and spirituality includes both historical and political elements. Only recently because of women working in the fields of historical, archaeological, and anthropological research, such as Merlin Stone and Marija Gimbutas, have we begun to learn of the pre-patriarchal history of Goddess-worshiping civilizations. Archaeologists and cultural anthropologists have brought to light this hidden and timely knowledge which can be used in clinical and religious settings to help women heal.

In Chapter 3, I present a psychospiritual perspective of healing founded in Goddess-based spirituality and feminist psychology. This chapter differs from many of the other chapters because it is concerned not only with individual healing but also with social and political change. It encourages women and men to acknowledge female spirituality and the power of the Goddess, and describes how this acknowledgment has the power to heal both men and women.

As a sexual abuse counselor in a community agency, I interviewed and treated a variety of women suffering from the results of rape and childhood sexual abuse. Their voices, stories, and healing bring structure and meaning to this chapter.

Chapter 3

Tales of the Goddess: Healing Metaphors for Women

Sharon G. Mijares

Goddess spirituality affirms both a woman's sexuality and body, and therefore promotes deeper healing. Women are in the midst of a rebirth, for during the past few decades a vast amount of evidence has been unearthed which illuminates the eras prior to the written historical accounts of humanity. Numerous religious icons have been found indicating that the female body was revered for its fertility and sexuality. A woman's menstrual cycle associated her with the movements of the moon and nature, creating a deep connection between women and the universe.

In ancient cultures the Goddess was associated with the planting and the harvesting of crops. Her body changed, seeds sprouted, and She was able to bring forth fruit. Humanity was in awe of the female, for women's bodies were similar to the Earth Goddess. These ancient civilizations passed on myths honoring their Goddesses. These Goddess narratives affirmed the power, sexuality, and beauty of women. The female was honored and divinely associated with the cycles of birth, death, transformation, and rebirth.

These early practices changed dramatically. Approximately 6,000 years ago female sexuality was denigrated with the onset of patriarchy. This change had a serious impact upon the relational, psychological, and spiritual well-being of humanity. Anthropologist Marija Gimbutas (1991) believes that prehistoric matriarchically governed societies lived in peace. In the middle of the twentieth century (1946), sociologist Violet Klein recorded that in pre-Christian times men had been dependent upon women economically. Women had managed the primary sources of income; they had been the owners of the homes, producers of food, and providers of shelter and security for others.

With the onset of patriarchal dominance, property rights shifted to men; women also became designated as property. As a result, current statistics from the 1997 United Nations high commissioner for human rights (Robinson, 1998) reveal that

> 70 percent of the 1.3 billion people living in poverty are women. The increasing poverty among women is linked to their unequal situation in the labor market, their treatment under social welfare systems and their status and power in the family. (p. 3)

Anthropological research, supported by sacred texts such as the Bible, reveals the onset of a dominant belief that it was a male's obligation to control female sexuality. Women's bodies became a vehicle for men's pleasure and control. Female sexuality was no longer revered and women lost control over their own bodies. Spirituality was separated from physical life, and sexuality became associated with lust and sin.

As a result, many women carry a considerable amount of shame about their bodies. It is probably true that the majority of women around the world do not accept the sacredness of their bodies and they certainly do not view the vaginal canal as a sacred passage into life. Many women are ashamed of their bodies and their sexuality. For example, many women will not look at their own bodies. They describe their bodies as "disgusting." This is particularly true of women who have been sexually abused.

When we examine the female population of this planet we learn that violence and sexual abuse are occurring throughout it (Gnanadason, 1993; Robinson, 1998). For example, in the United States statistics suggest that a woman is beaten every fifteen seconds, a rape occurs every six minutes, and one out of every three girls is sexually abused before her eighteenth birthday (Fortune, 1984). Much of this abuse is related to long-held beliefs that women should be subordinate to the male population. Physical violence injures the woman's spirit as well as her body. Violence against the body is violence against the soul.

Many of humanity's problems are centered in the rejection of our natural sexuality. This repressive influence may contribute to sadistic and aggressive impulses, including the excessive use of pornography and sexual abuse. We must relearn and obtain a healthy acceptance of natural eroticism and sexuality. Human sexuality and spirituality can be in positive relationship. The reemergence of the previously hidden history of Goddess spirituality offers opportunities for completing this needed healing (Eisler, 1988; Gadon, 1989; Stone, 1976). As a result of the unearthing of prehistoric evidence of Goddess-worshiping societies, women have begun an effort to restore their bodies, minds, and souls.

We cannot discuss women healing from abuse without understanding the role of the body and memory. Many massage therapists and other types of body therapists have found that cellular structures within the body release memories when manipulated. This is especially true of intense emotional memories. Although scientists have never claimed to find the specific location of the unconscious mind, somatic psychologists associate the unconscious mind with the body. The body is not a passive mechanism dominated by the brain's impulses, but rather a living system vibrating with feeling and an intelligence of its own (Damasio, 1999).

Previous beliefs determined that the brain controlled the body, but current findings in neuroendocrinology and the study of the enteric nervous system reveal that hormones and neurotransmitters are continually being transmitted between the body and the brain (Bergland, 1988; Gerson, Kirchgessner, and Wade, 1994; Rossi, 1993). Conversations are taking place between the brain and body-mind. Hormones travel through the bloodstream. Cells are listening and cells are speaking. Even though specific functions have a relationship to right and left brain hemispheres, there is no evidence of a place in the brain for yoga training and another for a dance lesson. Research on hormones and the enteric nervous system shows the message capabilities of the ovary and gut. These studies suggest that messages travel from the brain to the endocrine system and also from the endocrine system back to the brain (Bergland, 1988; Gerson, Kirchgessner, and Wade, 1994).

Archetypal energies are available to help women find healing and wholeness. Carl Jung and Joseph Campbell both believed that archetypal forces of the collective unconscious were manifested in our biology (Mijares, 1995, 1997). They are preconscious psychic structures containing biologically related patterns of behaviors—qualities and expressions of human life. States of consciousness exist at every level of our being. In the separation of mind and body we have been severed from a larger field of potential consciousness. Women by nature are more in touch with their bodies. For example, women have monthly menstrual cycles and the capacity to bear children. The fact that "mother" and "matter" come from the same root Latin word (meter) supports women's deeper relationships to physical life and the body.

Therefore a profound relationship exists between the demeaning of women and the separation of mind and body. This separation reflects a gender imbalance that affects all humanity. Its results are revealed in both religious history and in the denigration of the body. Women are essential in the process of healing this imbalance. To rebalance humanity, women need to acknowledge not only their feminine beauty but also their instinctual power.

Instinctual power is centered in the body. Many women are not grounded in their bodies. The ideal female portrayed by the media is unrealistic. Many advertisements contribute to distorted body perceptions, which often result in eating disorders among women. The average woman cannot compete with overly thin fashion models and glamorous Hollywood stars. A generation of young women is starving itself, attempting to follow these cultural icons. Is this what we want for our daughters, sisters, mothers, partners, and friends?

Many forms of sexual abuse exist. Cultural images do not offer enriching paradigms for young girls to emulate. Music videos often portray women as sex objects. It is conceivable that the suppression of women and the defamation of the body and sexuality have contributed much of the psychopathology manifesting in a variety of sexual perversions and sexual confusion. A 1995 U.S. postage stamp acknowledged the late Marilyn Monroe. The caption beneath her picture tells us to "hold on to the legend." What *legend* did Marilyn Monroe's life suggest? She was an abused child who grew up to be objectified for her sexuality alone. How many persons knew Marilyn's intimate feelings and values? In her loneliness and despair she committed suicide.

Feminine models that empower women by affirming our potentials, health, and wholeness are unequivocally needed in our culture today. Goddess spirituality grounds us in our bodies. It is a human necessity that we must reclaim this heritage. Both women and men can benefit by understanding the historical, religious, and evolutionary contributions to the psychological and spiritual difficulties of this age. This clarification can assist women's healing processes. We can observe how stories change and as a result acknowledge our own abilities to create new narratives that encourage psychospiritual healing and gender balance.

THE SPLITTING OF EARTH AND SKY

Over 3,000 years ago a significant change took place in humanity's psychological and spiritual evolution. The patriarchal model of social organization established dominant power. Patriarchal society is based upon a hierarchical system of government. Women, children, sexuality, the body, and the earth are not at the top of the list. Ancient Greek mythologies referenced a splitting between male and female, the mind and body. Prehistoric myths had announced the marriage of Earth and Sky, proclaiming this secured fertility as they were merged in sexual union. These cosmologies reflected the changes taking place on earth. The storytellers began to speak of the forced separation of Earth and Sky, resulting in the loss of their sacred union (Parrinder, 1971).

It is believed that these changing myths reflected the beginning and dominance of rationalization. As mental capacities heightened, the body's relevance was being negated. The rise of the patriarchal religious and philosophical social systems created a chasm between the cognitive-mind and body-mind. Women, matter, and form were relegated to an inferior position. Creation myths reflected these changes. For example, the Greek Goddess Athena was birthed out of the mind of her father, Zeus, and Eve was formed from Adam's rib.

Yet the earlier versions of these myths differ. The historian Merlin Stone (1976) explains that the goddess Athena was worshiped by the Mycenaeans long before the Acropolis of the Greek civilization was built. In fact, the temples of the Acropolis were built upon earlier Mycenaean foundations. Athena had existed as a goddess in her own right before the revision that now has her being born from the mind of Zeus. How many people know that Eve, the designated scapegoat for all human sin, was actually Adam's second wife? There are earlier myths that tell us about Lilith, Adam's first wife. Earlier stories also describe an alternative meaning to Eve's creation from Adam's rib (Barnstone, 1984; Stone, 1976).

Ancient Sumerian legends give us a very different version of Eve, and they also reveal that Eve was Adam's second wife. In Merlin Stone's historical text *When God Was a Woman* (1976), we learn of Lilith. In the original legends of the Sumerian Goddess Inanna, Lilith is proclaimed to be the "hand" of the Queen of Heaven. Lilith also appears in an ancient Hebrew legend as the first wife of Adam. In this myth she refuses "to lie beneath him" and flees. Lilith appears again in later Kabbalistic writings. In this version, the hand of the Goddess Inanna is now called a demon. It is said that, "Lilith, Queen of the demons, or the demons of her retinue, do their best to provoke men to sexual acts without benefit of a woman, their aim being to make themselves bodies from the lost seed" (Stone, 1976, p. 195). Much harm has been done from similar projections and irrational interpretations of male sexual fantasies, but we could not begin to understand this phenomena without the evolutionary development of psychological understanding occurring in this century.

Lilith was cast into alliance with the demons and her replacement, Eve, was formed from Adam's rib, or so we have been told. When we examine research (Kramer, 1963) on the early Sumerian myths we also learn of an earlier and very different version of Eve and the rib.

According to Sumerian scholar Samuel Noah Kramer (1963), an earlier version of the paradise legend takes place in Dilmun, the "land of the living," a land that is "pure" and "clean" and "bright" (p. 147). One of the Sumerian gods, Enki, the water god, notices that Dilmun has no water so he gets Utu, the sun god, to bring water up from the earth and Dilmun is "turned into a garden, green with fruit laden fields and meadows" (p. 148).

Kramer's telling of the rest of the Sumerian paradise myth casts further light on the later biblical version of Adam and Eve being cast from the Garden of Eden after eating the forbidden fruit. Kramer describes how Ninhursag, "the Great Mother-Goddess of the Sumerians" (1963, p. 148), causes eight special plants to grow in the garden. The plants thrive as a result of an "intricate process of three generations of goddesses" conceived by Enki and born "without the slightest pain or travail" (p. 148). Ninhursag does not want these plants eaten, but Enki eats them one by one and as a result Ninhursag condemns him to death. Soon Enki's health begins to fail and disease enters into eight of his organs—"One of Enki's sick organs is the rib" (Kramer, 1963, p. 149). The Mother-Goddess is finally persuaded to heal Enki and she seats Enki by her vulva. She births eight deities (one for each ailing body part) and they heal Enki's illnesses. His rib is healed by the goddess Nin-ti or "lady of the rib."

Cass Dalglish, a writer and translator who works with Sumerian women's stories (1996, 2000), points out that the pictographic sign used to tell this story is *ti,* sign number 73 in Rene Labat's (1976) lexicon. It is relevant to know that *ti* means both "to live" and "rib" (p. 69). This double meaning makes the story of healing of the rib by the "Lady of the rib" or the "Lady who makes live" (Kramer, 1963, p. 149) a great pun in Sumerian. In Kramer's words, "It was this, one of the most ancient of literary puns, which was carried over and perpetuated in the Biblical paradise story, although there, of course the pun loses its validity, since the Hebrew words for 'rib' and 'who makes live' have nothing in common" (p. 149). The play on words is lost in the language of the Bible.

Kramer (1963) points out the many similarities in the Sumerian garden of the Gods to the biblical paradise story. He explains that the poem describes this Sumerian paradise to be in Dilmun which is "a land somewhere to the east of Sumer," and suggests that

> there is good indications that the Biblical paradise, too, which is described as a garden planted eastward in Eden, from whose waters flow the four world rivers, including the Tigris and Euphrates, may have originally been identical with Dilmun, the Sumerian paradise-land. (Kramer, 1963, p. 148)

Kramer's scholarly renditions of these Sumerian texts give women a very different history. As many feminists writers have pointed out, the creation story becomes Eve's story.

The later translations of Eve's creation from Adam's rib appear quite different given the earlier Sumerian perspective. Later translations served to sublimate women. Making Eve the scapegoat for the loss of paradise and viewing the pain of childbirth as a curse has not encouraged respect for woman as the origin of all human life. Instead, the stories were rewritten to associate the female with weakness and mistakes. These later creation myths certainly did not elevate, allow for the equanimity of, or benefit women. Religious authorities told women that their role was to be submissive to the superior male. Social and cultural influences have continued to perpetuate this destructive narrative. These influences have contributed to the prevalence of rape and sexual abuse.

Lilith's refusal to lie in the "missionary position" during sexual intercourse is a metaphorical reference to historical changes taking place as patriarchal religions claimed domination over women and goddess spirituality. The sacred texts of religions and myths proclaimed the downfall of women. For example, the Zend-Avesta of the ancient Persian Zoroastrian tradition warned that a man would be put to death if he had sexual intercourse with a menstruating woman (Darmesterer and Mills, 1974). The Old Testament also expounded on menstrual and childbirth taboos and proclaimed male dominance over women. According to Deuteronomy 22:13-21 (*The Holy Bible,* King James Version) a husband had the right to stone his newly purchased wife if she was not a virgin. Riane Eisler (1988) notes that Leviticus 12 explains that "a woman who has given birth to a child must be ritually purified lest her 'uncleanliness' contaminate others" (pp. 101-102). Woman, once revered for her sexuality along with her capacity to give life, was reduced to the position of property; her innate ability to give birth became her shame.

Whereas woman and her natural capacity as birther of life were being reduced to an association with sin, man was now *conceptualizing* life from the abstract realms of the mind. Early Greek philosophers placed emphasis on truth and critical thinking, the "atomists" (Greek physicists) supported materialism, determinism, and reductionism; Plato gave attention to the form (the idea) behind all objects. The Greeks discovered and named the mental realm of abstract reasoning. More attention was given to the ideal than to the actual object. For example, the form (an ideal or conceptualization) received more respect than the actual embodied person. "Spirit" was greater than "matter." Sky and Earth had indeed split! Because women are by nature more related to matter, form, and birthing, they too were subdued.

The mystic-philosopher St. Augustine was a major influence in the development of Westernized Christianity. He was also deeply influenced by Platonic philosophy and likewise believed that spirituality was to be obtained through the use of the reasoning mind. Life was merely a symbolic representation giving us clues of an "invisible reality of God in heaven" (Leahey, 1987, p. 61). Faith was given greater importance than life itself. It was proposed that women, sexuality, and the body (including the Earth) distracted the male from his loftier ideals and aspirations. Therefore, women's role was to serve the male because he was closer to the Divine. In his text, *A History of Psychology,* Thomas Leahey (1987, p. 67) explains that

> Europe's antifeminist attitudes came from the Romans and even from Aristotle, who considered female infants as suffering from some sort of birth defect. Christianity, however, intensified the Classical [era's] disrespect for women, linking women to sexuality as the foundation of sin and temptation, and instituting a schizophrenic attitude toward good women (virgins) and ordinary women, who were at best mothers. As St. Thomas Aquinas said, "Woman was created to be man's helpmate, but her unique role is in conception . . . since for other purposes men would be better assisted by other men." (*A History of Psychology,* Second Edition, by Leahey, Thomas, ©. Reprinted by permission of Pearson Education, Inc., Upper Saddle River, NJ.)

This misogynist belief remained largely uncontested until the latter part of the twentieth century. Religion and philosophy have supported the negation of women (Gnanadason, 1993).

Early psychology made its own contributions. For example, the founder of psychoanalysis, Sigmund Freud (1856-1939), wrote a paper in 1923 asserting the primacy of the phallus for both sexes. Feminist psychoanalyst Karen Horney (1885-1952) argued against this theory, explaining that women yearned for the *advantages* in society ascribed solely to those who possessed penises, but that most women were likewise content in their inherent ability to bear and nurture new life from within their bodies (Fadiman and Frager, 1994).

Sigmund Freud believed that the human being was motivated by various impulses and instinctual drives. Libidinal energy was sexual in its nature, and manifested in our drives and desires to fulfill our human needs. Defense mechanisms were activated to protect the ego and also to prevent the natural flow of libido. According to Freud's theory the superego and the ego censored unacceptable psychic material. Patriarchy manifested this behavior in the external world by suppressing women and failing to acknowledge women's unique expression of embodied spirituality.

Hysteria was a widely used psychopathological diagnosis during Freud's time (Leahey, 1997). The word *hysteria* comes from a Greek word for womb. The Greek physicians blamed the ailment on a diseased uterus. This was a common diagnosis for women because it was believed that only women became hysterical. Perhaps this and similar diagnoses are related to more than 3,000 years of sexual repression, incest, and sexual abuse.

Freud and his colleague, Joseph Breuer, found that the cause of hysteria was repressed, traumatic memories. They believed that the symptoms manifesting from these repressed memories could be cured by expressing repressed feelings such as grief, rage, and terror. Freud, pressured by his colleagues, withdrew his proclamation that many women were suffering the effects of sexual abuse. He replaced this earlier finding with the Oedipal-Electra complex, based upon the ancient Greek myth of Oedipus, who unknowingly killed his father and married his mother. Freud's revised theory proclaimed that psychological distress was indicative of the repression of childhood sexual fantasies involving the opposite-sex parent. This complex was given preference; it was an easier answer than the closer examination into widespread sexual, religious, and cultural abuse of children and women would be.

More recently, this problem has reappeared in the form of the "false memory" debate. Defenders of the false memory theory debate the validity of memory retrieval. The American Medical Association (1994), American Psychiatric Association (1993), and American Psychological Association (1994) have acknowledged that a great deal of abuse occurs regularly and that abuse can be forgotten. It is also true that some psychotherapists have led clients to believe they were abused as children. But these debates have led people away from the more important issue. Instead of listening to the distress of women and the messages emerging from their bodies, researchers spend more time and effort debating the validity of the mind and its memories. Perhaps many of the unconfirmed false memories reflect the collective genetically transmitted experience of millions of women over the past few thousand years.

These sexual offenses to women are quite different from the experience of our ancestors who gave divine reverence to the female, her body, and her sexuality. In fact, 3,000 years of subservient and limiting identities for women have profoundly impacted our world. Both men and women have been very deeply influenced by the narratives passed on by their forefathers. Society has greatly suffered as the result.

The recovered myths of the prepatriarchal creation stories are helping many women to heal from a long cycle of abuse and negative self-narratives. These ancient global myths narrating the feminine as Goddess help reframe impoverished self-narratives and also offer encouragement for women healing from sexual abuse and other forms of trauma. As women retrieve this lost heritage they are empowered to work in relationship with other women and with men to heal families, communities, and the world.

As anthropologists and archaeologists continue to recover evidence of prehistoric Goddess-worshiping societies, humanity is being offered the potential to develop a new reverence for life and sexuality. Disrespect for the body and the Earth are likely related. Collectively, humanity is mutilating the earth by destroying rain forests, ravaging the land, and polluting natural resources. This is yet another form of violence against a material body. The split between Earth and Sky needs to be healed.

EMBODIED NARRATIVES

Only recently have we begun to understand these historical underpinnings which have contributed to the domination of women and children. Until the late twentieth century most women accepted feminine inferiority. How refreshing and healing it is to know that earlier creation stories affirmed rather than negated the feminine. Much is to be learned by studying ancient mythologies and the changes that occurred through the ages. Women can integrate this knowledge and use it to heal, for these ancient narratives proclaiming the power and beauty of the goddess have the power to heal both women and men.

There are many ways to retrieve this ancient wisdom. Professionals, students, and clients can read books by Riane Eisler, Marija Gimbutas, Merlin Stone, and other experts. Another method is experiencing a psychospiritual awakening through the knowledge released from within our bodies. Our bodies carry the memories of this ancient heritage, the acknowledgement of the divinity of women. These healing narratives are waiting to be evoked from body memory. If DNA can carry the information of how to build the human body, perhaps it also carries the memory of human experiences. Is it possible that universal myths are also biologically conveyed? Late mythologist Joseph Campbell believed this to be true (Mishlove, 1988). Carl Jung called this shared memory the collective unconscious. Both Jung and Campbell believed this memory was evidenced in the mythological narratives of all cultures throughout history (Jung, 1964; Campbell, 1949, 1974).

Archetypes are described as instinctive and universal elements of the unconscious mind manifesting from humanity's collective unconscious. These motivating psychic influences can include the common elements found in fairy tales, myths, novels, films, and our dreams. This includes psychic entities such as the masculine, feminine, warrior, magician, demon, sage, wise woman, Madonna, and divine child archetypes. This also includes the prehistoric memory of the great goddess and her many manifestations. The storytellers spoke of goddesses endowed with both grace and power.

The ancient Sumerian Goddess Inanna journeyed into the underworld (the unconscious), was killed by her dark sister, was resurrected through the intervention of dedicated friends, and returned to her queendom, empowered by the journey. The archetypal Hindu Goddess Kali Durga is associated with creation and destruction. This image of the power to create and destroy has been acceptable for masculine images of God, such as the Old Testament God, Jehovah. He both created and destroyed. Yet it has not been acceptable for women. Women were to be submissive, regardless of any abusive treatment. Religion, culture, and family life have perpetuated this limiting myth. The woman needs to know her shadow side in order to integrate instinctive energies. When archetypal memories of feminine power are evoked in a woman, she is well on her way to healing for she is reconnecting with elements of her instinctive body-soul.

These recollections can be used to free women from limited self-narratives by contributing to their wholeness. For example, there are many women whose femininity is very gentle and goodwilled, but they are unable to protect themselves from abuse by others. Women who are physically abused by their partners often remain in the abusive relationship because they "love him" and believe that their love will transform and end the violence. This ideal has rarely evinced healing in abusive relationships. Also, women who were subjected to incest or molestation as children are often emotionally vulnerable. Perhaps they repressed their rage at very young ages. Many adult victims of rape were also sexually victimized as children. The perpetrator recognizes their vulnerability and preys upon it. These women need to feel their rage.

Rage is a natural attribute meant to protect boundaries. It is linked with instinctive power. Getting in touch with this rage at a deep archetypal level doesn't mean that women need to act out violently. It empowers them to have a presence that dispels abuse by its very nature. This protective power is accessed from deep in the belly area of the body. Martial artists learn the centeredness required for their balance and skill, through breathing into the belly. Shamanic healers often access different powers through different centers in the body. This understanding can be applied to the myth of Inanna.

Inanna's sister, Ereshkigal, the Queen of the Underworld, killed her sister and felt no remorse. What does that mean? It is certainly against all of our finer values. First, Inanna had come to support her sister. Her act was based upon goodwill. She passed through seven gates (this could refer to the seven chakras, or energy centers, in the body) during her journey. At each gate she gives up something of value until at last she enters the realm of the Underworld (the deep unconscious depths within the body-mind).

This is one of our earliest stories reflecting a heroic journey. In Carolyn Edwards' (1991) version of the myth, Inanna's dark sister kills her with a glance. Perhaps Inanna saw the power of her dark side and it killed her limited self-image. After undergoing this death, Inanna was rescued by her friends and resurrected. Upon returning to her castle Inanna found her husband sitting on her throne wearing her garments and celebrating. With her newfound authority, she sent him to the Underworld. (The agreement upon her return from the underworld was that someone had to take her place.) Inanna had found the power to protect her boundaries. She demanded respect. No one had the right, not even her husband, to assume her throne. The throne represents her position (center) of power. Inanna makes sacrifices and manifests love for others but also learns to command respect. This is a story about balancing the opposites. Inanna becomes whole.

A psychotherapist can share this powerful story with a client. The listener may not cognitively understand its deeper meaning, but at embodied levels of the unconscious realms a response is initiated. The storyteller should read it slowly, creating a trancelike state of focused awareness. This metaphorical journey offers rich imagery to the unconscious mind and therefore deeper memories stir, memories of a time when women were honored. It reminds a woman that she needs to touch or be touched by the power of the shadow self in order to become whole. This story evokes something deeper from women's spiritual embodied memory leading to joy, healing, and wholeness. The following story applies this idea.

A woman entered therapy. She had been abused throughout her childhood and young adulthood. Similar to so many women who have been abused, she was not grounded in her body. The woman was continuously having relationship difficulties. She alternated between patterns of defensive behaviors and self-blame. Many of her significant relationships ended in discord. She couldn't figure out what she was doing wrong. After years of victimization due to personal boundary violations, she began to admit to her anger and also her desire for power. The woman experienced many boundary violations. She had to psychologically release herself from cultural and religious conditioning by acknowledging her desire for personal power and respect.

The denial of very old anger prevented her from feeling a sense of wholeness. She was angry that she'd been abused. In the healing process she recognized that an embodied sense of earthy, feminine power was a necessity. She had previously lacked a connection to instinctual and primal human nature. Knowledge of the goddess myths supported her healing process.

The word *power* strikes a chord of mistrust in many women; many people are afraid of it because of its long-term history of human misuse. This woman had reached a significant stage in her psychospiritual healing. She began to trust her own intuitions, senses, behaviors, and heart-inspired motivations. She had a few friends with troublesome, intrusive behaviors. Suddenly, the woman found herself unexpectedly and firmly protecting her boundaries. She simply but powerfully expressed her expectation for respect, and each of these intrusive women humbly complied. She didn't act out of anxiety, aggression, or manipulation, for her "truthfulness" was the expression of her power. At first, she was amazed at this embodied sense of authority. As she progressed in her healing, it became natural for her to expect others to give her the same respect that she gave them. The myth of the Goddess Inanna's entrance into the Underworld was very meaningful to her. She had been able to integrate the unconscious attributes alluded to in the story.

During this time the woman had also begun to value her body. She joined an athletic club and learned to be able to walk around the shower room naked with other women without shame. She began to feel the energy and strength in her body through aerobic classes, dance, and other forms of physical movement. Her healing became more complete as she integrated it into her body.

Physical movement and dance are very important healing tools for women. In this century we have seen the return of spirituality in body movement and dance thanks to pioneers such as Isadora Duncan and Ruth St. Denis (Miller, 1997). The healing process can be greatly enhanced by movement and dance. Although beautiful, ballet rarely allows for sensual movements of the hips or breasts. In ancient times women danced to honor their sexuality, fertility, connection to the earth, and the universe. Belly dancing honored female sensuality and helped prepare the body to birth babies through it's undulating movements. As a woman begins to reclaim her body, she also needs to experience the joy, beauty, and power of movement. Movement and dance bring mind and body together and also help ground these awakening energies.

Trance dancing, such as Roth and Loudin (1998) teach, allows a woman to experience embodied sensuality and power. Its unique beauty is in its primal expression. A woman's wholeness is dependent upon awakening her instinctive side. When a woman learns to use all of her body (which traditional ballet does not advocate) and to allow natural flowing movements, it encourages the development of instinctive intuition. In my experience even an aerobic dance class can encourage a woman to feel more embodied and whole. The more we recognize the inner wisdom of the body, the greater the opportunity for wholeness.

When a woman centers in her body (rather than her head), she begins to develop a grounded sense of authentic presence. Hatha yoga, Tai Chi, aikido, belly dancing, and other forms of fluidic movement are very therapeutic, grounding, and an integral part of the healing process. The potential for acknowledging one's strength, compassion, and wholeness is greatly enhanced. A focus on body awakening supports the emergence of archetypal and spiritual forces. As the body releases its chronic muscular locks, energies are able to flow through it. In this opening, heaven and earth intermingle. This experience supports the healing of the split between mind and body.

The goal of the entire healing journey is to know one's authentic nature, the greater Self. A woman has missed the point of the healing process if she gets stuck in her anger or views herself as a victim of the patriarchal system. A woman's most valuable attribute is her relationship with her authenticity.

A wonderful Japanese myth of the Great Mother Sun-Goddess, Amaterasu-Omikami, is paraphrased from *The Storyteller's Goddess* (Edwards, 1991):

> Amaterasu has a brother, Susanowo, who is jealous of her greater power. She hopes for the best, accepts his words of affection, and plans for a good future. He gets drunk, his anger grows, and destruction begins. In her frustration and despair

Amaterasu retreats to a cave and closes herself off from the world. The gods and goddesses cast Susanowo from heaven into the realm of darkness. The queendom is in despair without the light of the great Mother Sun, so the spirit of all living things begins to wither. They come up with a plan to stand outside the door to her cave holding pieces of shining mirror while using what strength they have left to sing and dance with joy in her honor. Amaterasu cracks open the door to the cave and her own beauty and radiance are reflected back to her by all the pieces of mirror. Needless to say, she returns to her place in the world.

When a young girl or woman has been abused, her spirit retreats and lives in isolation. Her authentic Self is no longer present and a coping personality takes its place. This story can facilitate the therapeutic emergence of a woman's power. The metaphor for power is enacted by the gods and goddesses who cast out Susanowo. They protect the boundaries of something great, metaphorically portrayed as Amaterasu. This myth can be used to evoke the woman's return to authentic life. The next step in the healing process will be for the woman to acknowledge innate radiance and to allow this radiance to manifest in her life. The following is another example of how this myth was used to help heal and empower a rape victim.

The woman was progressing in the sessions, acknowledging her feelings but still feeling the disempowerment caused by the rape experience. Having been trained in Ericksonian hypnosis and Stephen Gilligan's self relations psychotherapy, I find it natural to use the metaphors portrayed in the Goddess stories as they provide healing narratives. As with many women, her symptoms were related to low self-worth and an inability to fully connect with the relational field of life (Gilligan, 1987, 1997). I utilized the story in a trance as Amaterasu's brother is cast out (metaphorically representing the abuser) by the gods and goddesses (powerful support is available), all the little beings (connections to life) holding the pieces of mirror reflect (and remind) her of her authentic Self (beyond the abuse) and that it's safe for her to come back into life. The woman related to this story on unconscious and conscious levels. She soon returned to normal life. She was even feeling better about herself than she had before the rape.

THE CYCLES OF A WOMAN'S LIFE

Early Greek mythology teaches a woman about the various stages leading toward greater wholeness. Greek myths portrayed life as a heroic journey. They honored the different stages of a woman's aging process and created seasonal rituals that honored this initiatory journey. Many women have suffered because of the cultural loss of respect for the aging process. The first step is for the woman to recognize the gifts within each of these stages. The next step is to create rituals that enhance the journey.

When a woman learns to appreciate the various archetypal influences representing the maiden, mother, queen, and crone she can appreciate and accept the aging process. She will not need to attempt to create an illusion of youth through cosmetic surgeries. Greek mythology was rich with goddess rituals honoring the cycles of life. Regular rites were performed in honor of Demeter, both goddess and mother. Homage to Demeter assured the harvesting of crops and the birthing of children. Greek myths also spoke of the abduction and rape of her daughter Persephone by Hades, the god of the underworld. Persephone disappeared from earth as she was pulled into his realm. Demeter searched the world, lamenting for her daughter. Demeter's grief and wrath manifested in famine. Finally, she tricked Zeus into assuring the return of her daughter. As a result, spring returned. Once again the crops grew and the harvest was full.

Elinor Gadon (1989) explains that this "myth hinges on the violence of young women's sexual initiation and the wrenching separation from the protective mother, social realities of many women's lives under male domination" (p. 157). Persephone is also linked to Kore in the Homeric hymn. Kore represents the virgin, the untouched feminine self.

Persephone is the maiden; Demeter is the mother. These are two of the phases in the life cycle of a woman. A third archetypal of the feminine is called the crone or the wise old woman. In Greek mythology she was called Hecate. She appeared at significant times in the legends. This feminine triad represents very important archetypal aspects of the female journey; maiden, mother, and crone.

Recently, my friend Kamae Miller, editor of *Wisdom Comes Dancing* (1996), shared her theory concerning an additional aspect of the feminine cycle. She used the Arabic word *malika* to describe a queenly state that is beyond the mother and not yet a crone. This queenlike stage is more suitable in our time. Women over forty and younger than sixty-five may not identify with the archetypal influences of the maiden, mother, or crone. Perhaps this newly coined phrase allows for the emergence of the Self. In a culture that struggles against the aging process, the crone is not a welcome image. Women are longing for a deeper sense of identity, yet they are not sure what that means. In this queenly phase, the woman is self-contained. She has the bearing of beauty, compassion, and wisdom. The following client story illustrates the dynamics of these ancient archetypal forces in an aging woman's life.

Teresa, a divorced woman in her early fifties, came to me for psychotherapy because of deep anxiety and depression. She had just ended a brief affair with a much younger man. As this attractive woman told me her story, I recognized the power of the maiden archetype. She had not been able to secure an ongoing, satisfying relationship in her life; therefore, the maiden's desires remained unfulfilled. She was still motivated by the power of the maiden archetype, but its imbalance had brought her disappointment, emotional pain, and sexual abuse.

Men were always attracted to her strong mothering nature. Once a man was attracted to her, the mother archetype manifested in a desire to nurture him by sharing spiritual teachings and attempting to guide him in his life. Despite her good intentions, neither of these feminine expressions had been working very well for her, and she was in despair. She needed the wisdom of the older wise woman archetype to help her glean the learning obtained from successes and failures in relationship. The crone also manifested in her desire to share spiritual knowledge. This archetypal wisdom needed to be evoked more. The therapy session centered on this need. In meditation she experienced a glimpse of this older, wiser guide, yet she still shied away from this powerful archetype.

Within the month following this visual experience in therapy, she also manifested the first indications of the onset of menopause. She was afraid of aging. She acknowledged her concern that she may never have the loving relationship she had longed for, especially because men of all ages tend to pursue younger women rather than older ones. She was grieving. She was not ready to accept the power or cultural status of the crone at this transitional stage, but she was ready to hold the space for the emergence of the feminine Self within her. The therapy primarily consisted of goddess stories as my client breathed deeply to enhance a state of receptivity and unconscious response. In this trance state she experienced the beginnings of a transition as this queenly nature emerged.

A year after our last session this woman reported that she continued to feel more secure with her aging process. She felt more at peace with her life and her relationships. She shared that she was now comfortable with herself whether she was with other people or alone. This was a significant step for her to achieve.

There are many aging women at this crossroads. Their children are gone. They may be in a relationship or they may be single; but there is a sense of dissatisfaction and a longing for something more. They are ready for the next phase of their lives—the emergence of a greater Self.

RECLAIMING THE GARDEN OF PARADISE

Many women gather to share and to listen to stories of maiden, mother, queen, and crone. These mythological themes are included in individual psychotherapy and also in group rituals. Women need to talk about their wounds, including feelings about their bodies, their sexuality, and aging with other women. These issues can be the focus of individual psychotherapy with a feminist psychotherapist. Women can also receive healing benefits by joining a women's group (see Photo 3.1).

A feminist psychotherapist is not afraid to share her personal healing experiences. She does not dominate the client. They mutually discuss how the woman feels about her body, her sexuality, and her relationship to self and others. The woman's healing can then be enhanced by joining a women's group, particularly one that practices women's spirituality. As women bond and share their stories, they affirm a feminine way of being. The authentic Self is acknowledged and mirrored back to each participant. In this loving, empowering en-

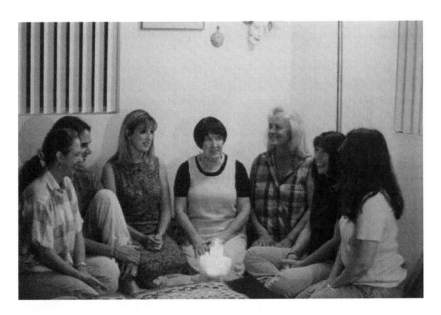

PHOTO 3.1. Women's Circle. Courtesy of Sharon Mijares and the North County Sacred Women's Circle.

vironment the women are able to affirm one another's experience. These personal narratives need to be listened to and acknowledged so that psychospiritual healing can occur. Women need to learn to trust each other. They are often confused about their feminine identity, as masculine models of behavior have dominated for almost 6,000 years.

Disclosure is encouraged. Each woman's experience is sacred because it is related to life on Earth. Spirituality and life are interrelated in goddess spirituality. During meetings, women may discuss intimate feelings. They can share their successes, acknowledge their hopes and fears for their families, and discuss social and environmental conditions. They also often share past wounds caused by sexual or physical abuse.

If statistics state that one of every three women was sexually abused before the age of eighteen (Fortune, 1984), then many women may need to bring these feelings into the circle. Lighting candles, burning incense, drumming, and creating ritual space provides a safe, integrative space in which each woman can talk about her painful sexual experiences. For many women, their first sexual experience as a girl or young woman was not a sacred event but rather a painful or shaming memory. Her story is shared in the circle. Each woman is asked to articulate what she needed at that time. She is then supported emotionally by the other women in the circle. During the ritual each woman can declare what she is releasing and then what she is claiming. The women's circle will affirm the inherent sacredness of each woman, her sexuality, and her body. Group participation enhances and grounds the experience. This type of a process replaces the tendency to get stuck in limited self-negating identities.

Drumming, storytelling, and dancing evoke ancient memories within women—memories of female ancestors gathering around fires to share their knowledge of childbearing, healing skills, and love. Similar rituals are also organized around the aging process. In most groups the women create rituals. Ritual enhances the depth of the experience and promotes healthy emotional integration. Author and psychotherapist Judith Duerk (1989) asks women:

> How might your life have been different if there had been a place for you, a place of women? A place where other women, somewhat older, had reached out to help you as you rooted yourself in the earth of the ancient feminine. . . . A place where there

was a deep understanding of the ways of women to nurture you in every season of your life. A place of women to help you measure your own stature . . . to help you prepare and know when you were ready.

A place where, after the fires were lighted, and the drumming, and the silence, you would claim, finally in your Naming, as you spoke slowly into that silence, that the time had come, full circle, for you, also, to reach out . . . reach out as younger women entered into that place . . . reach out to help them prepare as they struck root in that same timeless earth. How might your life be different? (p. 67)

Women have much to contribute at this time of our humanity's evolution. Women are becoming more in touch with their bodies and the Earth. As birthers of life they bring an enriched understanding of relationship. Goddess spirituality is rooted in the earth and human relationship. Earth and life itself are given reverence, for they are manifestations of the Divine. It is time for a more *embodied* relationship with life, for embodiment is one of the basic tenets of goddess spirituality. As women reclaim their spirits and their bodies, they can stand in partnership with men and in unison heal the planet and redeem humanity. This psychospiritual healing will also have a healing impact upon future generations. In this work of love, harmony, and beauty, heaven (sky) and earth will be reunited.

REFERENCES

American Medical Association (1994). American medical association council on scientific affairs. Report on memories of childhood abuse. Chicago, IL: Author.

American Psychiatric Association (1993). Statement on memories of sexual abuse. Washington, DC: American Psychiatric Association.

American Psychological Association (1994). Working group on investigation of memories of childhood abuse. Interim report. Washington, DC: Author.

Barnstone, W. (Ed.) (1984). *The Other Bible: Ancient Alternative Scriptures.* New York: HarperCollins.

Bergland, R. (1988). *The Fabric of Mind.* New York: Viking.

Campbell, J. (1949). *The Hero with a Thousand Faces.* Princeton, NJ: Princeton University Press.

Campbell, J. (1974). *The Mythic Image.* Princeton, NJ: Princeton University Press.

Dalglish, C. (1996). Moist Wind from the North. Dissertation novel and companion essay submitted to The Union Institute, Cincinnati, Ohio. UMI 9623650. Ann Arbor, MI: UMI.

Dalglish, C. (2000). *Nin.* Duluth, MN: Spinsters Ink.

Damasio, A. (1999). *The Feeling of What Happens: Body and Emotion in the Making of Consciousness.* New York: Harcourt and Brace.

Darmesterer, James and Mills, L. H. (1974). *Zend-Avesta.* New York: Gordon Press.

Duerk, J. (1989). *Circle of Stones.* San Diego, CA: LuraMedia.

Edwards, Carolyn McVickar (1991). *The Storyteller's Goddess.* San Francisco: HarperCollins.

Eisler, R. (1988). *The Chalice and the Blade.* San Francisco: HarperCollins.

Fadiman, J. and Frager, R. (1994). *Personality and Personal Growth,* Third Edition. New York: Harper and Row.

Gadon, E. W. (1989). *The Once and Future Goddess.* San Francisco: Harper and Row.

Gerson, M. D., Kirchgessner, A. L., and Wade, P. R. (1994). Functional anatomy of the enteric nervous system. In Leonard R. Johnson (Ed.), *Physiology of the Gastrointestinal Tract,* Third Edition (pp. 381-422). New York: Raven Press.

Gilligan, S. (1987). *Therapeutic Trances.* New York: Brunner/Mazel, Inc.

Gilligan, S. (1997). *The Courage to Love.* New York: W.W. Norton and Company.

Gimbutas, Marija (1991). *The Language of the Goddess.* San Francisco: HarperCollins.

Gnanadason, Aruna (1993). *No Longer a Secret: The Church and Violence Against Women.* Geneva, Switzerland: WCC Publications, World Council of Churches.

The Holy Bible, King James Version (n.d.). London: Cambridge University Press.

Jung, C. J. (1964). *Man and His Symbols.* New York: Doubleday and Co., Inc.

Klein, V. (1946). *The Feminine Character.* London: Routledge and Kegan Paul.

Kramer, S. (1963). *The Sumerians.* Chicago: University of Chicago Press.

LaBat, Rene. (n.d.). *Manuel D'Epigraphie Akkadienne (Signes, Syullabaire, Ideogrammes).* Paris: Librairie Orientaliste Paul Geuthner, S.A.

Leahey, T. H. (1997). *A History of Psychology: Main Currents in Psychological Thought.* New Jersey: Prentice-Hall, Inc.

Mijares, S. (1995). Fragmented Self, Archetypal Forces, and the Embodied Mind. Doctoral dissertation. UMI 9608330. Ann Arbor, MI: UMI.

Mijares, S. (1997). Narratives and neural winds. *Somatics: The Journal of Mind-Body Arts and Sciences.* Winter: 22-25.

Miller, Kamae A. (Ed.) (1996). *Wisdom Comes Dancing: Selected Writings of Ruth St. Denis.* Seattle: PeaceWorks.

Mishlove, J. (1988). Conversations on the Leading Edge of Knowledge. Understanding Mythology with Joseph Campbell. *Thinking Allowed.* Video series #S075. Oakland, CA: Thinking Allowed Productions.

Parrinder, G. (Ed.) (1971). *World Religions: From Ancient History to the Present.* New York: Facts on File Publications.

Robinson, Mary (1998). All Human Rights for All: Fiftieth Anniversary of the Universal Declaration of Human Rights 1948-1995. Geneva: United Nations High Commissioner for Human Rights, No. 2, 3.

Rossi, E. (1993). *The Psychobiology of Mind Body Healing,* Second Edition. New York: W.W. Norton and Company, Inc.

Roth, G. and Loudin, G. (1998). *Maps to Ecstacy: A Healing Journey for the Untamed Spirit,* Revised Edition. New World Lib.

Stone, Merlin (1976). *When God Was a Woman.* New York: Harcourt, Brace, and Jovanovich.

JUDAISM

One of the most beautiful creation stories from the wisdom traditions is found in Judaism. The following version of *tzimtzum,* a Jewish creation story, demonstrates the relationship of psychological and spiritual healing. Rabbi Strassfeld narrates (Strassfeld, 2002) the psychospiritual work to be discovered and experienced in the human journey.

How did the world begin? For Jewish mystics the world began with an act of withdrawal. God did *tzimtzum.* God contracted God's self to leave space for the world to exist. Before that God was everywhere, filling every space and every dimension. After this *tzimtzum*—this withdrawal—some divine energy entered the emerging world, but this divine light, this divine energy was too strong, overpowering the worlds that tried to contain it, and the universe exploded with a cosmic bang. Shards of divine lights, of holiness, were scattered everywhere in the universe. The sparks of holiness are often buried deep in the cosmic muck of the universe, they are difficult to behold and yet they are everywhere, in everyone, in every situation. They are the life and meaning of the universe.

We live in this world of shattering. We feel in our bodies and in our souls the brokenness of the world. We too feel at times the resonance in our selves of that initial cosmic shattering. Our bodies, like that primordial world, try not to contain, but rather to hold onto the divine light and energy flowing around us and in us. But, as in the world's origin, our bodies are too frail, made only frailer with the passage of time, and so we begin to leak our divine image/energy. Perhaps then illness is really leaking of our souls. In this world of shattered hopes and expectations, we search for wholeness.

Moses, as you know, shattered the first set of tablets, the first set of the Ten Commandments. And then he got a second set that he helped to write. When the Ark was constructed for the sanctuary, the rabbis tell us not only the whole second set of tablets was put into the Holy Ark, but the pieces of the first set as well.

Wholeness comes not from ignoring the broken pieces, or hoping to magically glue them back together. The shattered co-exists with the whole, the divine is to be found amidst the darkest depths and the heaviest muck of the universe. Every moment has the potential for redemption and wholeness. Our brokenness gives us that vision and the potential to return some of the divine sparks scattered in the world. (p. 500)

In his chapter on Jewish methods for psychological and spiritual healing, Sheldon Kramer shares Jewish Kabbalistic teachings and healing practices. His chapter illustrates Jewish ways for healing psychological wounding that are founded in the Kabbalistic Tree of Life teachings. The chapter also portrays the meaningfulness of Jewish holidays and rituals as a system of individual and community development. Dr. Kramer's chapter is filled with practical examples of ways to heal our everyday human encounters with self and others.

Chapter 4

Jewish Spiritual Pathways for Growth and Healing

Sheldon Z. Kramer

INTRODUCTION

Jewish spiritual pathways are based in the Old Testament (Torah) or what is known as the Five Books of Moses. Traditionally, the Torah is studied in four ways. The first involves reading the literal story; the second looks at the biblical stories as a metaphor; the third involves reading the stories and understanding the spiritual laws that govern human nature and morality; and the fourth is the secret dimension or what is called the mystical perspective. This fourth dimension is least understood in Judaism even though it has been part of Judaism since the beginning of monotheism. The father of monotheism, Abraham, is considered the first Jewish mystic. He was interested in natural law and the process of creation. Abraham would often commune with nature. Through his positive encounters with G-d, he was able to carve a profound pathway to help humanity evolve.

One can view the Old Testament as a story of a group of people that are chosen to reflect the spiritual laws found in nature. Their outer journeys were fraught with human frailty, resulting in rebelliousness and alienation from natural law. The story demonstrates the consequences for becoming out of harmony with this natural growth process.

What is not very well known in Judaism is that connected to the mystical dimension are writings of the Kabbalah (meaning "to receive," in Hebrew). These writings show how to clarify pathways for inner guidance, to teach methods to transform consciousness, and also to guide our actions in everyday life. These writings came from the original Jewish mystics known as the *nisterim* ("hidden ones"), also known as Kabbalists. They were responsible for the mystical interpretations of the creation story found in Genesis in the Old Testament of the Bible. This chapter focuses on Kabbalistic concepts and methods. It demonstrates how these teachings are used to heal psychological discord and spiritual deprivation. The mystical dimension can be integrated into everyday life when one follows an inner and outer discipline reflecting these teachings. This endeavor will lead to a more peaceful and happier life.

KABBALISTIC PATHS OF HEALING

Creative Sparks

According to the Genesis story in the Old Testament, human beings are made in the image of G-d. This of course means that we have tremendous creative potential within ourselves. We can learn to focus our minds and utilize these creative energies in order to manifest what we need and want in our daily lives. The Jewish mystics meditated. This illuminated state enabled them to directly understand the creative forces existing both within us and manifesting in the outer world. Through deep contemplation of this creative energy field, the mystics of yore understood that in the beginning there was invisible energy without end. (In Hebrew this is called *Ain Sof.*) This invisible energy was found within the darkness. The Kabbalists called it "the lamp of darkness" because it contained this unseen creative light.

> Since the creator was everything, it was all-one and by itself (a-lone). Because it was one, it meant that the Creator was all by itself. The Creator's wish was to create form from its formless energy state. This occurred because this Creative Intelligence wanted to give of itself. This energy without end's first manifestation was light. This light was called in Hebrew, *Or Ain Sof* (endless light). Everywhere was this powerful endless light that was full of abundant energy. *Or Ain Sof* contracted a pinhole of darkness in the center of itself. In this darkness *Or Ain Sof* placed a sliver of light. It took this action to have mercy on the visible creation that was about to be manifested. The light had compassion for the creation; it would have been too powerful for more than a sliver of light to enter this vacuum. When the

sliver of light was put into the darkness, a volatile movement of nine contractions took place. These contractions were caused by the contrast between the light and darkness. Vessels were formed to hold this light. When this endless light contracted and expanded, the mystics received the vision of these ten lost vessels, which became arranged in the shape of a tree. (Kaplan, 1998)

It is believed that Abraham wrote the Book of Creation *(Sefer Yetzihrah)*, the first text in the Tree of Life teachings (Kaplan, 1988). This chapter will focus on these particular Tree of Life teachings because they offer practical methods for developing congruency with the different aspects of oneself. This includes the ability to think, feel, and act with impeccability. When our thoughts, emotions, and actions are aligned, a unification occurs which facilitates contact with our spiritual core nature.

The hidden mystical interpretation of the Book of Genesis as described in Kabbalah stated that these ten energy intelligences, called *spherot* of the Tree of Life, consist of unity *(keter)*, wisdom *(chochmah)*, understanding *(binah)*, love *(chesed)*, strength and discernment *(gevurah)*, compassion/inner beauty *(tiferet)*, dominion *(netzach)*, receptivity *(hod)*, stability *(yesod)*, and kingdom, a word pertaining to responsibility, faith, and humility *(malchut)*.

The ancient lost Tree of Life teachings comprising the ten faces *(spherot)* of G-d reflect our own many faces. These qualities can be said to be balanced archetypes found within the psyche. Our journey is to connect with these archetypes, which were the divine sparks for humanity. The mystics knew that their vision of fragmented sparks contained the map for returning to internal balance. That was the secret: the Tree of Life can reconnect us to pathways between the sparks within ourselves. It reminds us of the work we need to do toward reunifying ourselves.

BALANCING YOURSELF
ON THE TREE OF YOUR LIFE

The ancient icon of the Tree of Life is a natural map of the human body (see Figure 4.1). Just as trees do, we also have roots: our feet are planted on the ground. We have a trunk and spinal cord running through the center of us, similar to the sturdy center of a tree. We have

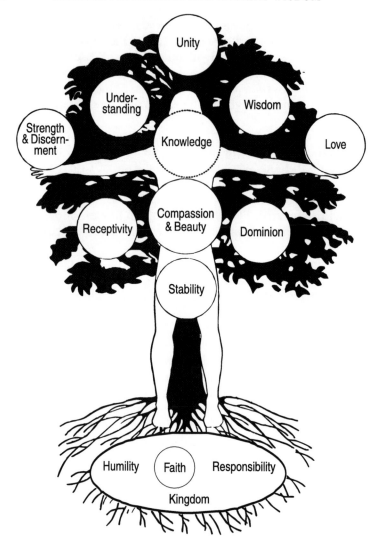

FIGURE 4.1. Tree of Life. Courtesy of Sheldon Kramer.
Note: Person in figure is facing the tree.

lower branches—the lower limbs of our body. Our arms, branches, stem from our trunk, and our heads form the upper parts of our branches reaching the crown of our heads. This is similar to the crown of the tree, which is connected to the sky and heavens above us.

At the bottom of the Tree of Life is the *spherot* of *malchut,* translated from Hebrew as "kingdom." This place, located below our feet, is where we take responsibility every day to walk our own path on the Earth. It is the interaction between our bodies and how we maneuver in the outside world to get our basic needs met. To successfully survive and become responsible in everyday life we must have faith that our roots and the earth will sustain and nurture us, not only through the food we eat and the shelter we receive from the natural products that we utilize but also in the world of relationships. Relationships help us to maneuver inwardly and outwardly in our everyday lives. To be rooted or anchored in our lives, we must have a belief or trust in something greater than ourselves. This foundation helps us live to in meaningful ways. Basic trust in life profoundly affects us. It is experienced first at an early age from the mother or other caregivers as they interact with the young infant.

Having faith in life is one of the most important attributes of human life. We need to embrace feelings of hope and to believe in new possibilities for our futures. Without this positive frame of mind, we would not be motivated to continue to act in responsible ways. We each need to feel that some light exists at the end of our own individual tunnels. Most human beings are blocked in some way in that imbalance is often not recognized. We all have dark shadow sides of ourselves. Our task is to find balance in our lives.

Many people lack a basic sense of trust in the world, mainly because wounding has occurred in their relationships. Because of this woundedness, many people seek psychological healing.

Edith recently consulted with me because she had an exacerbation of her chronic pain. She was also experiencing chronic fatigue that was connected to a recently newly diagnosed condition called fibromyalgia, which is chronic pain and tension in the muscles. As I listened to the history of her relationships, I learned that she had experienced early child abuse by her brother. She had been married three times; each man was abusive. She tended to be a caretaker, yet she partnered with independent, hostile men. Edith is caught in this pattern because of her lack of trust in the universe. She did not believe she could have nurturing men in her life, nor was she inwardly open to receiving this gift. This evidenced her basic lack of faith in the powers of the earth to provide what she needed and closed her to the possibility of receiving goodness in her environment. When persons lack this basic foundational trust, their spiritual belief in a Higher Power existing within and beyond this planet is limited. Inwardly they do not believe that anything or anyone is available to help them achieve what they need in everyday life. This is the root that needs reverent healing in Edith's foundation of life.

In the following discourse, we will move upward from branch to branch on all the *spherots* of the Tree of Life. This means symbolically understanding the teachings from right and left sides, the middle, and all the way up to the top of it. We will examine how this understanding is used to help Edith to heal and to balance her life.

The Tree of Life can be divided into three parts. The right side represents expansive energies, and the left side, contracting ones. The middle trunk moving to its roots is considered the balancing point between the opposites. In Kabbalistic methods for psychotherapy we maneuver between the right and left sides of our own tree and work on the synthesis of these two energies. Our purpose is to achieve the ultimate balance in everyday life. We also want to balance giving and receiving on all levels. The lower branches of the Tree of Life are connected to action. These branches are found directly above the roots. The right-hand side is the giving aspect of ourselves. The left side is our ability to receive or take from life, including others.

Edith predominantly resides on the right side of her lower branches, as she tends to be a caretaker. She does all the giving. In this role her previous husbands eventually abused her. This pattern led to her divorces. Currently, she was in a relationship with a boyfriend who was extremely pleasant and easygoing. However, he was very demanding of her attention. Her unmet needs dominated her life. Her caretaking was often not reciprocated because of her difficulty in receiving positive nurturance from others. The needed balance would come by focusing on the left side of the tree where she would learn how to take and receive from others. This brought up early childhood foundational issues because her parents, who raised her, abandoned and abused her, and her brother also abused her. The expectations of further pain blocked the energy in this branch related to taking and receiving.

A large portion of Edith's psychotherapy was focused on finding a needed balance between her positive giving nature and her ability to find reciprocity in her relationships. This included teaching her methods for monitoring her behaviors (left side, lower branch) related to receiving. On the Tree of Life paradigm, this balance of giving and receiving allows oneself to remain in the lower middle trunk and find the quality of stability (in Hebrew, *yesod*).

The Tree of Life locates this center of stability below the navel and above the genitals. The back and forth movements during sexual intercourse between male and female reflect the energy of giving and receiving. This helps humanity continue to procreate and to create stability within the human species. Without our need for sex, human beings would not naturally perpetuate the species. The Creative Intelligence of the Universe needs human beings to maintain its creation. People are the arms and hands of G-d. It is also meaningful that martial arts and other self-defense teachers usually emphasize focusing upon the navel, our stomach area, as it helps us anchor to the ground. This grounding centers us, facilitating protection from possible attack. People who have a difficult time finding and maintaining the balance between giving and receiving often manifest stomach problems. This appeared to be true about Edith as she also had colitis.

Balancing love with strength (middle branches) is another important attribute of wholeness illustrated on the Tree of Life. As our basic needs are met in the world of action, and we have some faith and hope about the future and getting our needs met, we feel more satisfied inside. This means becoming less defensive and being more open to emotional growth. We also become more receptive to others. We have the capacity to grow emotionally. In the Tree of Life teachings, the emotional qualities that we need to work on is the *spherot* of love and kindness on the right side of our chests, located in the right chamber of our hearts and right shoulder and arm, counterbalanced with the left shoulder point, left arm and hand with the left chamber of our hearts which is called the Spherot of strength.

Love is another expansive quality that has an enduring positive force. Love is attached to genuinely caring about oneself and others. This love is stronger than romantic love; it manifests from a selflessness truly desiring to serve others. The desire to help another person blossom is love for love's sake. It comes from an unconditional sense of giving.

In the case of Edith, she was extremely loving, pleasant, and easygoing. When she gave of herself to husbands and boyfriends, they demanded more. They also lost their balance in this energy exchange. Their response to her giving was to increase their possessive and dominating behaviors. This created a great deal of anxiety and depression in Edith, exacerbating her chronic pain and asthma. It is interesting to note that when one feels smothered in a relationship, one's breathing can also be affected.

To balance love we need to discern when to say yes and no to our emotional needs. This is embraced by the *spherot* of *gevurah* (left middle branch), which means in Hebrew "strength and discernment." It is also connected to the quality of creating boundaries and distinction in counterbalance to loving energy, which knows no boundaries. Edith's current boyfriend did not respect her boundaries. Both of them needed to establish appropriate boundaries, each in their own way. They struggled, as they were both out of balance. The balance between love and strength is the quality of compassion. This is connected to the *spherot* of *tiferet,* which in Hebrew means "compassion and inner beauty." When a balance between love and strength is developed, the inner beauty found within the heart shines through. People are often afraid that they will lose their ability to love if they focus on building inner strength. However, this development has the opposite effect. If strength is not coupled with love, it will result in imbalances within oneself and impair relationships. Blending and balancing these qualities is the essential work of the Tree of Life teachings.

The next task is balancing our upper branches of knowledge on the Tree of Life. On the right side we have the quality of wisdom—in Hebrew, *chokmah*—and on the left side we have the quality of understanding—in Hebrew, *binah.* The bridging and balancing of these two qualities lead to true knowledge or, in Hebrew, *daat.*

Consider what was happening with Edith in relationship to the upper branches. Edith tended to be overly analytic on the left side of her branches of the Tree of Life. She did not trust her intuitive sense or "sixth sense" to guide in her in relationships. Intuition would have helped her realize the need for appropriate boundaries. By focusing within and accessing her inner sense of what was needed she could have made the necessary shifts. Instead, she focused primarily on the left side of the upper branches of the Tree of Life as she attempted to analyze each problematic circumstance. The continuous mulling over and desperate search for answers often led her into ambivalence about her relationship. She needed to access her sixth sense. This inner knowing would guide her when to say yes and when to say no, and also when to have good judgment in terms of how to pick nurturing partners. As she worked on herself from this perspective, she was able to liberate the different energies and to begin to trust herself more. This shift in inner and outer perspective will lead to more peaceful interactions with herself as well as others.

When clients understand the human growth process as illustrated in the Tree of Life teachings, they do not judge their life circumstances as psychopathological. Instead, they enter into a spiritually meaningful process that offers an ongoing dedication to one's psychological healing and spiritual development.

THE THREE STRANDS OF THE SOUL

Nefesh

The Zohar (Book of Radiance), a Kabbalistic book, depicts what is called the "three strands of the soul" (Kramer, 1998). The Kabbalists utilized the image of the candle flame to demarcate the three main parts of ourselves. The lower flame connected to the wick and wax is connected to the *nefesh* (animal soul). This light flickers back and forth and is in the process of change. This corresponds to Freud's idea of the three parts of our personality, which he called the id, ego, and superego. (Id is our sexual and aggressive drives; superego is our social conscience; and ego is the mechanism that mediates between the id and the superego.) Contained within the ego are what are called in psychology subpersonalities. These subpersonalities are usually reflective of imbalances of the archetypes of the Tree of Life. For example, a subpersonality such as the "poor-me victim" is an aspect that believes everybody is more powerful than we are. We often feel similar to the child who is being abused by others. When we attach ourselves to this part we retreat from the environment or become angry and lash out because of our perception of being hurt—both animal-like instincts. The imbalance is becoming too receptive (lower left branch).

Similar to the candle flame, we are pushed around by these identifications and we separate from the different parts of ourselves (Assagioli, 1965). Another subpersonality is the "internal critic," who believes something is always wrong with him or her. The critic can always find fault in oneself and others (this imbalance is depicted by the left middle branch of discernment turning to criticism). The whole world is viewed in terms of how we or others are not living up to our expectations. A more extreme identification of this subpersonality occurs when the "critic" is the "dictator" who becomes a "bully" toward others and doesn't respect the wishes of others. Often the dictator/critical person tends to find others who are victims of their need for control. This is often found in dysfunctional, close intimate relationships.

Another subpersonality part could be called the "internal professor." A person such as this feels they are always teaching others from an intellectual standpoint. These people who have overidentified with this part of their mind often can't let their heart respond spontaneously to any human encounter. The world becomes kind of a unidimensional, emotionally dry place where one tends to feel alone and cut off from others.

Many other subpersonalities exist, such as the "frightened child," the "hypochondriac," the "silly one," the "guru," etc. All of these parts and the ones described previously are simply different aspects of our conditioning. They usually reflect early family-of-origin patterns that we learned as we interacted within our family environment. These aspects are brought to bear by external situations in the environment or by our internal thinking process. They are fueled by a variety of inner desires activated at one time or another. We are all looking for a relief from being overidentified with these different aspects of ourselves so we can have more internal freedom to act the way we want to be. In modern psychology, psychologists can often help someone adjust to different aspects of their personality. However, ancient systems of spirituality such as Kabbalah and the Tree of Life offer techniques for balancing ourselves by becoming more detached from our suffering. It is interesting to note that the Buddha himself often said the cause of suffering is attachment to things. We often attach ourselves to our own misery. This could be viewed as a type of fixation that limits our perspective. The Kabbalah and Tree of Life teachings, similar to concepts in Buddhism, show us direct pathways within ourselves to stand back from these kinds of identifications that push us around. This training in detachment is depicted by the next level of the flame (Assagioli, 1965).

Ruach

Located directly above the black and blue light is a steady yellow glow in the center of the candle flame. This part of the flame is called *ruach* (in Hebrew, "the divine wind, breath, or spirit"). The *ruach* has the ability to stand outside the *nefesh* and observe. It is the eye of the hurricane or a steady calm within the turbulence. From this perspective we can examine our tendencies to align with one particular personality self while ignoring other interior voices and needs. This illuminating clarity enables us to make choices.

Neshamah

Directly above this yellow glow is another filmy piece of light, called *neshamah* (suprasoul or higher self). The *neshamah* is that aspect of our psyche that is the unifying center. When we have successfully worked with the *nefesh* and *ruach* we are more receptive to this illuminating self. It can be viewed as a catalyst that participates in all the other reactions in the lower strands but tends to stand outside them. A useful metaphor found in the Zohar is that of *neshamah* being a prism; it is a catalyst for pure white light to bend itself into a multitude of pure colors that represent the different attributes of the branches of the Tree of Life.

The Unifying Agent

In working with the three strands of the soul, it is important to observe oneself in relationship to one's actions *(nefesh),* emotions *(ruach),* and thinking *(neshamah).* When we are more aligned with these functions, our *nefesh, ruach,* and *neshamah* are also aligned and we tap into the hidden fourth part, which is our spiritual aspect. This is the unifying agent among all of these internal centers. In meditation we access our *ruach* and *neshamah.* This becomes the main vehicle for achieving disidentification from different personality entrapments, for we now know the sacred within us. Our meditations help us reach this unveiling.

MEDITATION AND THE TREE OF LIFE

Many people are unaware of the contemplative meditation methods that are at the heart of Jewish spirituality (Kaplan, 1990). These methods are similar to other forms of meditational systems, such as *vipassana* found in Buddhism, *yoga* in Hinduism, or *zikr* in Sufism.

One Kabbalistic-oriented meditation practice that can be incorporated into psychotherapy is to directly utilize archetypal imagery, such as the candle flame in the description of the three strands of the soul, to help facilitate an altered state that transcends the variety of personality identifications and often creates in the meditator a deep relaxation response. The Three Strands of the Soul exercise is as follows:

> The meditator gently closes his or her eyes and visualizes a large flame. The tip of the flame should be visualized above the head. The practitioner should imagine that the yellow glow in the middle of the flame is within the heart (in the middle of the chest). The black and blue flame is in the pelvis. It is his or her own eternal flame of the Tree of Life. He or she is instructed to sense this image in the body. As the image deepens and strengthens, the meditator then begins to focus on deep, slow breathing, consciously inhaling and exhaling through the nostrils.

In the section that follows, I describe methods for integrating the use of meditation and Kabbalah that incorporate the use of a variety of breathing techniques and also use structured, guided, and spontaneous imagery (Assagioli, 1973; Kramer, 1998; Kramer and Mitchell, 2000).

The general method of Kabbalistic-oriented meditation is to contemplate a particular attribute that one needs to foster in one's own personal growth and development. Through active thought and imagery, one can imagine he or she is embodying this particular image in his or her life.

After determining which quality on the Tree of Life needs to be emphasized, the guide asks the person to follow the instructions for the Three Strands of the Soul meditation (as previously explained) to center himself or herself. Then he or she should articulate the quality needed for greater balance: for example, the quality of strength. Then he or she should imagine what that quality resembles in the imagination. The next step is to identify with the image and sense it in the body. Oftentimes this meditation encourages an inner experience.

Sylvia, who had recently ended her twenty-year marriage, was able to image, and feel greater strength as, a poised dancer. When contacting this image, she was able to feel the free spiritedness of her inner dancer. She burst into laughter and began to feel a sense of exhilaration radiating up and down her spine (the trunk of her tree) as she experienced joy! She used this image daily to help her gain increased self-discipline and self-confidence.

However, other persons doing the same integrative meditation and psychotherapy process might encounter resistances in both mind and body. The famous Kabbalist, Rabbi Nachman of Breslov, the historical famous Hasidic master, was psychologically minded. He recommended having a conversation with G-d when one is unable to actualize a desire. Nachman would advise followers to speak from the heart with the most sincere and deepest feeling possible, addressing the highest power of the universe (Kramer and Mitchell, 2000).

Often people ignore or block their deepest pain. When people sincerely open up to their highest power and allow it to enter this place of woundedness, the opportunity for healing is quickened. It can become a transformative attribute empowering their lives. Often lodged in these cathartic experiences are deep narcissistic injuries to the self that were the result of having abusive and neglectful parents. These generational patterns (Kramer, 1995) of imbedded suffering are then passed on as they continue to manifest in the relationships between parents and their children.

It is said in the Torah that the sins (imbalanced behaviors) of the previous generations are found within the youngest generation. It also says that if people choose to follow these commandments, they can be liberated from these particular fetters of the past. This statement is easier said than done. However, if we are able to attend to this core pain transmitted from one generation to another, we can truly liberate not only ourselves but the different aspects of the intra-generational legacy found within each individual. The healing of the generations from within is very much part of the process of returning to one's divinity. The following case example illustrates this belief.

When Vicki would try to meditate on the expansive quality of love, all she experienced was inner constriction. She easily and spontaneously expressed her unresolved hatred toward her mother. Vicki could easily access images of her grandmother yelling at her own mother. To help her resolve her feelings, she was guided to initiate a creative dialogue between her internalized grandmother and her mother to resolve the internal pain she experienced because of their hurtful behaviors. This helped her release fear, anger, and grief. During a following episode Vicki saw how her mother was repeating what had been done to her. The continued dialogue allowed for reunification and forgiveness. As greater compassion ensued in Vicki's inner family, she was able to receive love.

My books, *Transforming the Inner and Outer Family* (1995) and *Hidden Faces of the Soul: Ten Secrets for Mind-Body Healing from Kabbalah's Lost Tree of Life* (2000), elaborate these healing processes.

RETURNING TO YOUR SOUL:
THE RELATIONSHIP BETWEEN RABBI AND STUDENT

The close relationship between teachers (in Judaism, rabbis) and their students has been a longtime tradition in Hasidic circles. Hasidic masters are often not only teachers but also guides and advisors. They will help individuals assess and work on their personal *tikkun* (self-rectification). They often are healers for both individuals and the community. According to the Kabbalistic tradition, the only way one can be truly spiritual is to enter into the *tikkun* process. This is the work of polishing and refining one's personality attributes in order to reflect the universal balance of the different archetypal personalities of the Creator. Guidance is needed to complete this work.

This relationship between teacher and student borders on friendship. Often the student is invited to the teacher's house for special dinners. It might be at sundown on a Friday night to celebrate the twenty-four hours of sacredness of the Sabbath. Often the teacher and students will gather and celebrate in a joyous fashion, or one can choose to work deeply within oneself in a meditative fashion.

Psychotherapy, by its very structure, is a one-way relationship with strict boundaries. In some ways, it is an artificial relationship that doesn't allow a genuine two-way interchange. A rabbi has more flexibility than a psychologist to form a real relationship with his or her student. The rabbi may become an idealized good parent that one never had growing up who prescribes specific ways of living better. The rabbi becomes a model that the student can directly observe. This, of course, doesn't happen with psychotherapists.

A rabbi is not trained in psychopathology. When a person's needs are too overwhelming for a rabbi, a referral to a mental health professional for further assessment may be necessary. A rabbi is not trained in the methods of healing the deeply embedded wounds of the psyche; here the rabbi's role is limited.

People with more severe psychological disorders need extra help. Intense spiritual work may create more stress on an already unstable personality. Therefore, a spiritually oriented approach such as those found in the deeper Kabbalistic practices may not be useful. The results are blocked by the severity of the disorder. Psychotherapy might prove to be more appropriately applied at this time. However, some people may find it beneficial to return to traditional Judaism, with its many outer rituals and practices, to help organize their psychological stress (see pp. 114-119, this text).

COMMUNITY AS HEALER

The Jewish spiritual path is very community oriented. The rabbis will facilitate individuals, couples, and families to belong to this greater community. In fact, many troubled individuals often turn to rabbis in the community to regain a feeling of self-identify and connectedness to others. Many rabbis will encourage and invite individuals to religious services to facilitate a community context. In some religious communities, some people are taken into shelters where they can heal from their difficulties. Programs have been created for people who are drug and alcohol dependent. Because these programs focus on Judaism as a specific, particular path for spiritual growth, they differ from traditional twelve-step programs that focus on nonspecific spiritual paths.

Judaism has a natural holistic perspective. It has both an inner and outer dimension focused on individual and community relationship. It combines internal growth and outer ritual. One does not necessarily have to be a "religious" person to work on psychological and spiritual development; however, for certain individuals, the best healing that can take place is to be involved in a religious practice connected with traditional Judaism, which would differ from the deeper meditative processes. Some people are not ready for meditative-type exercises. Meditation and other relaxation procedures have an effect of letting go of internal tensions and worries. Some people actually need to hold onto this state of mind and body, otherwise they would possibly encounter a deeper level of trauma that they are not ready to face. Sometimes meditation exercises can increase anxiety and depression.

People who experience more extreme anxiety and depressive states are those who may benefit from more outer religious practices found in traditional Judaism. Orthodox Jews tend to follow the Torah in fundamental ways. They follow the written law and are committed to prayers and festival regimens. I have found that many people with tremendous anxiety or depression are helped by these outer activities, for they deemphasize the individual's personal difficulties and refocus them toward something greater. The refocusing includes spiritual study, as well as doing good deeds in the community. The rich rituals associated with Jewish holidays support a strong sense of Jewish community spirit.

JEWISH HOLIDAYS: HOLISTIC DAYS

One of the unique aspects of the Jewish spiritual path is that throughout the calendar year there are many holidays that the serious-minded spiritual ardents in this tradition could use to accomplish self-growth. The holidays follow the different seasonal solstices and are imbued with a great deal of psychological and spiritual meaning that can help an individual obtain psychological balance. There are many major and minor holidays that one could follow throughout the year. In each of these major Holy Days, it is commanded in the Old Testament to take off time from one's usual work. Traditionally, this would mean perhaps going to services at the synagogue or spending time with one's immediate and extended family. If the practitioner takes these holidays seriously, there is opportunity for deep meditation and a focus for working on self-transformation. In the following sections, some of the holidays are briefly described. How practitioners can work on themselves to achieve freedom from internal psychological disturbance is also discussed.

The High Holidays: Rosh Hashana and Yom Kippur

Jewish festivals follow the lunar calendar. The beginning of the year occurs usually in early fall in September. *Rosh* in Hebrew means "the head"; *hashana* in Hebrew means "the year." It is the celebration of the Jewish New Year. This is symbolically a time for self-renewal and for celebrating the birth of G-d's will. One can view this as the Creator's birthday when the Earth was born. This holiday reflects the story of creation found in Genesis. It is the holiday to reinforce one's faith and to trust in the world and the natural laws that govern it. As one follows the prayers and meditations, one is imbued with new hope that the year will bring "good" things, especially if you follow the path of Torah.

This is a time to reflect on oneself and to examine the deeds of the previous year. It is interesting to note that the English word *sin* usually has a negative connotation in Western religions, especially in traditional Judaism and Christianity. Many people think that sinning means you are a "bad person." In the original Hebrew in the language of Aramaic, *sin* means to "miss the mark." Similar to an archer trying to hit bulls-eye, the archer can miss hitting that center goal. The center goal in life is to achieve balance according to the ancient mystical teachings of Kabbalah. Rosh Hashana is a time to focus on our deeds that missed the mark and perhaps caused ourselves or others harm. At this time we try to look as objectively as we can at our actions of the previous year.

In following the spiritual path there are meditations that one can follow which can help one achieve this increasing self-awareness that is so important in psychological healing. For example, we can sit quietly, focusing on our breathing to relax while imaging a television screen in front of us. The next step is to literally go back starting from the here and now in the month one is in and then follow each week back throughout the past year. This is an important practice for people who take this meditation seriously to purge themselves from the emotional aftermath of turbulence that occurred throughout the previous year.

The Ten Days of Awe

There are ten days between Rosh Hashana and another holiday called Yom Kippur. Why ten? Once again, ten is a mystical number and goes back to the Ten Commandments, as well as being connected to the ten energy intelligences that were previously described on the Tree of Life. Each day corresponds symbolically to one of the ten *spherot*. Kabbalists focus on the quality for each successive day. They meditate deeply on the previous year, examining when they were in or out of balance with each of these qualities in their various life experiences. They then visualize and determine how to best work on perfecting these areas of holy attributes during the next year. Many religious people take time off during this period and view these ten days as an important preparation for Yom Kippur, which is the day for letting go of accumulated negativity. In fact, some religious Jews who are very spiritually oriented take off a month before Yom Kippur to achieve this kind of increased self-awareness in preparation for letting go of the previous year's disappointments.

Yom Kippur

The traditional way to describe Yom Kippur is the Day of Atonement. Although if you break this word down into the various parts it is really the day of "at-one-ment!" In other words, if you atone your "sins," considering those actions that were off balance or had missed their mark from the previous year, you can then help restore yourself to wholeness or "at-one-ness."

Yom Kippur day is the most solemn day of the year. It is a time to confess to G-d one's sins toward others, as well as sins against G-d himself. Spiritually you are literally instructed to unburden your soul in front of the Creator. It is time to cry like a child in front of one's parents for what one has done in an imbalanced and wrong way. In fact, many people go to other people that they have potentially hurt that previous year and apologize, as well as ask them for forgiveness to help clear any misunderstandings or wrongdoings. It is interesting to note that in traditional twelve-step programs, making amends is also a part of the recovery process. During prayer services, many of the melodies are solemn and allow a person to weep. Through weeping, the body softens and the mind wakes up. There is a sense of self-renewal. This particular method of operating at this time of the high holidays reflects psychological principles found in intensive psychotherapy. Most psychotherapy is aimed ultimately at letting go of fear, anger, and grief to help encourage expression of repressed or suppressed emotions so one can return to wholeness.

The Festival of Chanukah: From Inner Darkness to Light

The holiday of Chanukah falls on and around the winter solstice. This holiday commemorates the Jewish people historically winning a battle against all odds. This holiday symbolizes victory over oppression of outward religious freedom. On Chanukah, one can also examine how to overcome psychological oppression (parts of ourselves that limit us and cause disturbances in our relationships). The other part of this work is finding the courage within to work on those aspects of our lives. The mystical dimension of Chanukah is symbolic as a reminder that even in the hibernating winter months there are always new possibilities in the future. Hibernation is similar to sleeping, for there are always available life-giving forces to be accessed in the darkness. To restate it more simply, in the darkness there is always light! Carl Jung acknowledged that the dark unconscious contained unknown possibilities waiting to manifest into the light of consciousness. As mentioned before in the Kabbalistic doctrine of the Tree of Life, the darkness called *Ain Sof* is invisible energy without end—it is also called the lamp of darkness. During the holiday time, candles are lit representing the eight days of Chanukah. Each night we are commanded to recognize the miracles that are abundant around us to give forth hope in the future. Miracles are to be considered abundant and received directly from the infinite. Chanukah is celebrated in eight days. The mystical interpretation of this is that eight is the symbol of the infinite. If you turn the number eight on its side, it is an infinite symbol. In the original story of Chanukah, a flask of oil was found in the destroyed temple after the fierce battle was won. This flask of oil, which provided light, was supposed to last only one day; instead, it lasted eight days.

Passover: A Time for Personal Renewal

Passover is another major holiday, this time centered around the spring solstice. It corresponds with the Christian holiday of Easter. It is a holiday filled with symbolic meaning. Spring brings new possibilities and hope for harvesting new potentials. This holiday focuses on the Jews being externally enslaved by the Pharaoh of Egypt. However, the inner meaning of the holiday metaphorically teaches us that we need to know to free ourselves from the enslavement of internal addictions or difficulties. The holiday, similar to Chanukah, psychologically reminds us of those things that oppress us internally, but it also offers inspiration to work on rebalancing ourselves. This will enable us to bear better and more ripe fruit in the future.

Many symbolic foods are prepared for this holiday. One of the most important foods is called the bread of affliction, matzah. This comes from the story of the Old Testament when the Jews rushed to flee Egypt. They did not have time to allow the bread to rise before baking. Symbolically, unleavened bread is very thin bread to remind us to keep the quality of humility in abeyance. Leavened bread has an expansive quality to it and corresponds to pride and boastfulness. As we all know, feelings of superiority toward others and about ourselves can throw us off balance and lead to poor relationships. The matzah is a constant reminder that we must remain humble; through humility we can remain balanced and lead a peaceful life. It is also a reminder to continue to have better faith in oneself and others, as well as in the Highest Power of the universe.

Shavuot: A Remembrance of Spiritual Revelation

Shavuot is the festival commemorating the deliverance of the Ten Commandments that Moses channeled from his illuminating contact at Mount Sinai. Between the holiday of Passover and Shavuot there is a forty-nine-day period of intensive work one does on oneself to prepare for the spiritual revelation similar to what Moses experienced on Mount Sinai. Why forty-nine days? Forty-nine is the amount of years Jews spent in the desert before they received the revelation. Forty-nine also corresponds to the seven lower *spherot* described in the Tree of Life paradigm, which are love, strength, compassion, dominion, receptivity, stability, and responsibility through faith and humility.

These seven attributes are reflective of G-d's sacred attributes. If we can purify ourselves during these forty-nine days, it is possible to taste the Divine by identifying with G-d and with the archetype of Moses that is in the collective unconscious of all Jewish people's minds. For example, the first week of Shavuot examines the quality of love. During that week people begin to meditate on the quality of love and start with each of the other qualities and integrate them with this love. For example, on the first day we meditate on the first attribute, which is love meditating on the manifestation of love itself. The second day we meditate on the strength found in love; the third day, the compassion of love; the fourth day, the dominion in love; the fifth day, the receptivity in love; the sixth day, stability in love; and finally, the last day, the responsibility in love. This process helps to integrate these qualities and strengthen the manifestation of love.

The second week focuses on the quality of strength; each of the attributes is blended with strength and so on until we reach the forty-ninth day. If we really work on this and observe ourselves during the day with these different qualities, we experience the nuances from inside ourselves and our relationships potentially improved. The fiftieth day, which is the blending of all the other forty-nine days, is the festival of Shavuot. At this point, we are said to be more purified in our minds and hearts and in a more receptive place to go more deeply in our meditation to realize the holiness of this day. We can be divinely inspired with hope for the future.

There are many other holidays; however, the ones discussed are the most important with which to work on ourselves spiritually. The holidays themselves are imbued with psychological meaning available to each person who wants to follow an in-depth spiritual odyssey of self-growth.

FUTURE DIRECTIONS IN JEWISH SPIRITUALITY AND PSYCHOLOGICAL GROWTH

The integration of ancient Kabbalistic concepts such as the Tree of Life teachings with meditation practices is only beginning to be renewed. Traditional rabbinic training has not really delved into these methodologies to help improve the congregation's internal spiritual lives.

Many people, especially younger ones, have left Judaism to follow other spiritual paths because they found specific methodologies for the transformation of consciousness, such as in Buddhist meditation or yoga. However, as can be seen in this chapter, there is a possibility to integrate both the inner and outer dimensions of the Jewish path and to be simultaneously connected through a community that reflects one's cultural roots. This is an important aspect of one's spirituality; many Americans find themselves denouncing or avoiding their Western roots and pursue spirituality in a Buddhist or Hindu context, which is incongruous with their personal background. This can be problematic when one develops intimate relationships and starts a family. How do we raise a child in the context of Buddhism when our cultural identity is not reflective in that domain? However, many spiritually oriented Jewish people who had left the tradition and embraced Eastern religions are returning, but are integrating the wisdom of Jewish spirituality with the wisdom of the East.

Many books are emerging that reflect this kind of cross-culturalization of different paths, especially in the Buddhist world. In his book *The Jew in the Lotus* (1995), Roger Kamenetz provides a detailed description of a group of rabbis who were asked to go to India to visit the Dalai Lama in order to help the Tibetans understand how the Jews survived the experience of being exiled. The Dalai Lama is concerned with preservation of the Tibetan traditions because Tibetans have experienced an exile similar to that of the Jews.

A slowly growing community of Jewish spiritually oriented people are re-creating some of these ancient Kabbalistic traditions under the mentorship of the internationally known Rabbi Zalman Schacter, who is considered the father of a movement called Jewish Spiritual Renewal. Jewish meditation centers are flourishing in different parts of the world (see Photo 4.1). Many different kinds of Kabbalistic books for both Jewish and non-Jewish readers are available of late. This phenomenon reflects the growing interest in the integration of Jewish spirituality into everyday life, as well as the potential appreciation of how different spiritual paths are connected together. The integration of Eastern and Western mystical traditions is truly a way for everyone to understand the universality of all religion and psychological and spiritual paths from ancient times. The realization of the commonality of these practices truly reflects the work for all of us to realize in this new millennium!

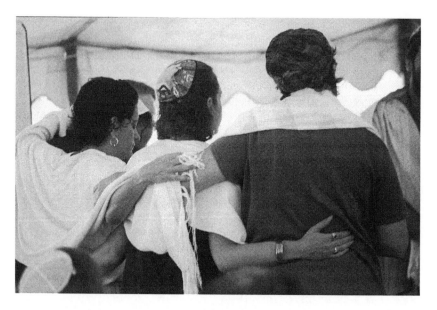

PHOTO 4.1. Jewish Renewal Meeting at Elat Chayyim where participants integrate inner meditations with an outer community that embraces the Jewish tradition. Courtesy of Rona Chayah Conrad and Elat Chayyim.

SUMMARY

Jewish spirituality and growth are based in the ancient lessons of the Kabbalah's Tree of Life teachings. The Tree of Life is a symbol of balance and can be used as a map to show where we need to rectify our personalities to achieve alignment among our *nefesh, ruach,* and *neshamah* (actions, emotions, mind, and spirit). When we achieve this alignment, we create the possibility of being able to receive the light of the creative energies in ourselves that reflects the unified energetic field. Jewish spirituality is considered both an inner and outer discipline and is best guided through a teacher who is connected to an established community that can help spiritual seekers ground themselves through psychological and spiritual growth in everyday life.

There are many outer holidays on the Jewish path. Jewish people create sacred space in honor of these holidays by taking time off from their everyday life to work on themselves psychologically and spiritually. These holidays contain rituals that offer both psychological and spiritual healing. The many Jewish rituals contribute to building a strong community. This is needed in our society considering its current fragmented, discordant nature.

The teachings of the Kabbalah offer psychological healing that is lasting and fulfilling; they connect us to the source and meaning of life. Much of modern psychology focuses on adjusting to life's never-ending dilemmas. Spiritual psychology, such as the teachings in this chapter on the Tree of Life as well as other transpersonal psychotherapies, aims at something more than "adjustment." Spiritually oriented psychotherapies offer means for defining our value systems. These teachings offer pathways that liberate us from imbalanced responses to life experiences. The unique contribution of the Kabbalah and Tree of Life teachings is that they ground spiritual experience in everyday life. In these teachings, one cannot live spiritually without simultaneously working on personality change.

REFERENCES

Assagioli, R.(1965). *Psychosynthesis.* Baltimore, MD: Penguin Books, Inc.
Assagioli, R. (1973). *The Act of Will.* Baltimore, MD: Penguin Books, Inc.
Kamenetz, R. (1995). *The Jew in the Lotus.* San Francisco: HarperSanFrancisco.

Kaplan, A. (1988). *Meditation and Kabbalah.* York Beach, ME: Samuel Weiser.
Kaplan, A. (1990). *Inner Space.* New York: Mozaim Publishing Corporation.
Kramer, S. (1995). *Transforming the Inner and Outer Family: Humanistic and Spiritual Approaches to Mind-Body Systems Therapy.* Binghamton, NY: The Haworth Press.
Kramer, S. (1998). Jewish Meditation: Healing Ourselves and Our Relationships. In E. Hoffman (Ed.), *Opening the Inner Gates: New Dimensions in Kabbalah and Psychology.* New York: Four Winds Press.
Kramer, S. (2000). *Hidden Faces of the Soul: Ten Secrets for Mind-Body Healing from Kabbalah's Lost Tree of Life.* Boston: Adams Media Corp.
Strassfeld, M. (2002). *A Book of Life: Embracing Judaism As a Spiritual Practice.* New York: Schocken Books.

NATIVE AMERICAN PSYCHOSPIRITUALITY

Native American traditions recognize the relevance of ritual for society. Rituals honoring the medicine wheel, pipe ceremonies, circle dances, sweat lodges, powwows, and storytelling help heal and bond the community. These traditions combine to give the individual a sense of place and purpose.

In their chapter on Native American psychospirituality, Terry Tafoya (a Taos Pueblo and Warm Springs Indian) and Nick Kouris demonstrate the use of storytelling and its significance for both individual and community healing. Storytelling is a primary element of the many Native American tribes, known as the First Nations' peoples. The stories passed on by our ancestors through oral tradition offer guidance for the human journey. They illuminate patterns inherent in the human experience. They evolved out of, and in turn serve to nurture, a deep connection with the land, elements, rhythms of nature, community, and the self—weaving a sacred web in which every individual was at once his or her own center and connected inextricably to the whole. This manifests itself in daily life, as spirituality is borne out of the art of living, providing context for the range of human emotion, and offering a path for growth.

When we consider the history of America and its effect upon the First Nations' peoples, it is not difficult to understand why alcoholism, AIDS, and despair exist in these communities. These communities have suffered tremendous loss, as we all have. One great loss is that the majority of humanity is disconnected from the most vital and sustaining aspects of life, Spirit and Mother Earth. Prior to the influence of Westernized culture, First Nations' peoples experienced a deeply rooted connection to both. Many psychotherapeutic programs, such as St. Norbert Foundation's Selkirk Healing Centre in Selkirk, Manitoba, and Thunder Child Treatment Center in Sheridan, Wyoming, use traditional Native American rituals to help First Nations' peoples recover from despair by reclaiming their spiritual foundation.

Native traditions teach us how to live in harmony with the Earth rather than destroy it. Americans have much to learn from First Nations' peoples and the land that we share. This learning will contribute to building healthy communities in order to survive the challenges of this era.

Chapter 5

Dancing the Circle: Native American Concepts of Healing

Terry Tafoya
Nick Kouris

INTRODUCTION

Stories are a form of medicine. They have the power to heal and to clarify identity. Stories also unify the community by reinforcing our cultural and spiritual continuity. Some stories carry a poison that deteriorates the spirit of the individual and the culture. The only difference between medicine and poison is the dosage. How strong is the dose and how much was ingested? There are many stories that teach us about these different expressions of power.

One such story of power is that of Cinderella—not the Walt Disney version, but the older, darker version of the legend. The two stepsisters can't fit their feet into the glass slipper, so their mother intervenes. One daughter is told to cut off her toes, the other daughter to cut off her heel. She then tells the emissaries of the prince to shove the bloody stumps of their feet into the glass slipper. This story helped to establish a frightening pattern of recognition for many American children. They grew up with the message there was only one way to be a "good member" of society—the falsehood of living a model that would never benefit the majority of its citizens.

To be a good American meant to be male, Caucasian, and Christian, to speak English as your first and only language, and to be heterosexual. Also, a good American obtained a certain level of education and income. The message was clear: If you don't meet these criteria, then you are to slice off whatever doesn't belong. You slice off your language, your sexuality, your gender—whatever doesn't fit.

Psychotherapists see many people who have turned to alcohol and other drugs, including high-risk sexual behaviors, as a form of anesthetic in an attempt to numb the terrible pain of this amputation.

Many of our high-risk clients and patients feel themselves to be "dismembered"—ripped asunder into disconnected parts of oneself. The opposite of the word *dismember,* as Susan Griffin (1992) points out, is the word *remember.* The stories we tell and encourage others to tell (which is ultimately what therapy and support groups are all about) help people to "remember" who they are, to allow them to become whole again. In the Indo-European roots of English, the word *heal* is related to the word *whole,* which is itself related to the word *holy.* This brings us back to the truth that stories (as so many people of the First Nations have said) are a form of medicine. With this in mind, let us begin with another kind of story (Tafoya, 1990).

EAST: NEW BEGINNINGS

Long, long ago, when mountains were the size of salmon eggs, and the sun still shone without embarrassment, there was a young woman about to be tied to the moon who was what we call in our language, *Ai-yai-yesh,* which would roughly translate into English as "stupid." Day after day and all day long, she would sit underneath the Cedar Tree and watch the world go by. Other young people her age would help their Old People clean salmon. These young people would help their Old People dig roots. They would help their Old People pick berries and tan deer hides. But not the Ai-yai-yesh Girl, she would just sit underneath the Cedar Tree watching the world go by.

Finally, one day, the Cedar Tree spoke to her. Now it may be that in the Old Days trees used to speak to human people a lot more than they do now, or maybe it's just that people used to listen a lot better than they do now. But the Cedar Tree said, "Ah, you're so Ai-yai-yesh—all you do is do sit underneath me. Watch, and I'm going to show you how to do something." Just so, the Cedar Tree taught her how to sew the roots of the Cedar Tree into circles. Circles are very important to many Native people. We are taught that the world is a circle, and the circle is the symbol for reciprocal relationships. One must give as well as receive and receive as well as give. Black Elk, the Lakota holy man, once said (Neihardt, 1961) that the wind, when it moves at its strongest power, moves in a circle.

As the young woman sewed these circles together, she wove the very first hard root cedar basket. Now, these baskets are very important to many Native people of the Pacific Northwest. Long ago, before white people came and brought Teflon, Tupperware, and microwave ovens, these baskets were one of the primary ways in which Native people cooked their food. The baskets were so well made that they could hold water. Hot rocks were heated in the fire and dropped into the water of the basket, which would make the water boil. But one had to keep stirring the rocks around, or the rocks would burn a hole through the bottom of the basket. One would feel really fine absorbed in the work. When Ai-yai-yesh had finished the basket, the Cedar Tree inspected it, and said, "You've done a good job, but your basket isn't finished yet, because it's naked. It has no patterns, no designs. A basket is not truly finished if it has no patterns."

She began to cry, and said, "But I don't know any designs."

"Ah, you're so Ai-yai-yesh," said the Cedar Tree. "Start walking—and keep your eyes and your ears and your heart open, and you'll find all sorts of patterns you can use."

So she began walking. But as she was walking she was crying, so she wasn't watching where she was going. This is another characteristic of Ai-yai-yesh people. Thus it was that she almost stepped on Wax-push, the rattlesnake. "And what's the matter with you, almost stepping on innocent people?" he asked, for rattlesnakes had bad tempers in those days too.

"I'm so sorry," said the young woman. "The Cedar Tree said if I just kept walking I'd find all sorts of patterns to use for my basket, but I haven't found a single one."

"Ah, you're so Ai-yai-yesh," the rattlesnake said. "You look at me—what do you see?"

So she looked at him—really looked at him. She found that if she looked at Wax-push in a certain way, the snake had diamond-shaped patterns all down the center of its back.

"Oh, what a beautiful design you are," she said.

"Take it! Use it for your basket," the rattlesnake said. And just so, she had the very first design for her basket.

She learned to weave the pattern of the rattlesnake into her baskets, and she was very proud of herself. Soon she started thinking, "I can't keep using the same pattern over and over again." She started crying again.

Someone else spoke to her, and this someone had a voice like thunder. "WHY ARE YOU CRYING, LITTLE GIRL?" It was Patu talking to her. The name *Patu* means "mountain"; it was the mountain talking to her.

She said, "I'm crying because the Cedar Tree told me if I only kept walking, I'd find all sorts of patterns for my baskets, but I've found only one."

Patu, the mountain, replied, "AH, YOU'RE SO AI-YAI-YESH! YOU LOOK AT ME—WHAT DO YOU SEE?"

So she looked—really looked at the mountain, and she saw that a mountain is indeed a triangle. "What a beautiful design you are!"

"TAKE IT! USE IT FOR YOUR BASKET," said Patu.

She now had another pattern. Everywhere she walked other things would talk to her and teach her. She saw the stars come out at night and form constellations she could duplicate. She saw the tracks of little birds, the shape of leaves, the designs of feathers, patterns on butterfly wings, and the shape of salmon gills. Everywhere, in all directions, there were all sorts of patterns she could use for her baskets.

When she had learned to put all these designs into her baskets, she returned home to her community, where she taught all of her friends and relatives how to make these baskets and how to put all these designs into them. And when she had done that, she wasn't Ai-yai-yesh anymore. *Ana-kush-nai* [the story is over].

Over the winter season, from the time the first frost is on the ground until the thunderstorms begin, stories such as this (a traditional story of the Sahaptin people) have been told within Native communities. The meanings of these stories are as complicated as many of the designs within the baskets. Although some anthropologists might term this legend the "Origin of Baskets" story, on another level the legend is about patterns of interactional behavior. On her healing journey, the Ai-yai-yesh Girl must discover there are many alternative patterns of behavior possible. This is one of the reasons that she realizes she can't keep using the same pattern over and over again. Indeed, one definition of pathology might be using the same pattern in all situations, without thinking about it. As in many traditional stories, the Ai-yai-yesh Girl teaches audiences to look to these legends as a model, a road map, of how to live one's life. In fact, stories serve the important function of metaphoric models that operate on many levels of awareness to teach what is proper and appropriate behavior. Stories both entertain and instruct the listener.

One of the reasons a number of Native Nations work with the concept of the "sacred hoop" or "medicine wheel" is to emphasize the idea that one's life is to be seen as a type of healing journey, no different than that of the Ai-yai-yesh Girl. The healing journey is ultimately related to accepting one's wholeness. (Remember that the words *heal, whole,* and *holy* all come from the same linguistic root.) There are predictable "signposts" upon the journey that one can anticipate, representing the four cardinal points of that Sacred Hoop. Indeed, there are times that one may feel Ai-yai-yesh—alone and isolated from one's community. Stories weave the individual into the universal; they speak to the permanence of lived experience.

The first direction might be seen as the direction of the East: the dawn, a new beginning, when something happens to challenge one's life. In the case of the Ai-yai-yesh Girl, it was when she realized she could not sit under the tree any longer. This may be a time for some people to realize they can't continue in the life they've been living. There comes a time when one makes a choice to walk this way or that.

In the Ai-yai-yesh Girl story, there is an archetypal initiation. It involves the movement from one level of awareness to another and the realization that more than one reality is possible. The eyes open and suddenly one sees a pattern: the diamond-shaped design of the rattlesnake, the triangle of the mountain.

In a similar vein, the tradition of the Katchina Dancers of the Hopi people of the American Southwest also serves as a vehicle for metacognitive learning. Before their initiation, Hopi children are taught that the Katchina Dancers are literally real. They are supernatural beings who embody a wide range of powers and temperaments. Indeed, the Katchina Dolls originally made to give to the children were intended as mnemonic devices to help identify the various Katchinas.

When the Katchina Dancers perform for the children and the community, the children are not privy to the knowledge that their relatives are actually the ones dancing behind the ceremonial masks. When the children are ultimately told during their formal initiation that the Katchina Dancers were their own relatives all along, they are given switches and told to flog the dancers. This instruction allows for a direct method to express anger and outrage at being lied to through a ritual that permits a charged emotional release, without the danger of the anger being internalized or directed against the community (Beck, Walters, and Francisco, 1977).

Many Native people tend not to express anger because it is seen as a type of spiritual pollution, a kind of energy that is harmful. If enough of the spiritual pollution clings to the spirit body of a human, it results in lowered resistance and can be one of the causal explanations of sickness. Among the Hopi, it is believed that the Katchina dislike public displays of anger. If they are offended, they refuse to bring rain. In a desert culture, this can mean death. It is therefore a considerable cognitive dissonance when the children are provoked and then publicly ordered to openly display their anger toward the Katchina Dancers. This is similar to the concept of "crisis" in the Chinese language: it is represented in the combination of two symbols— one represents danger and the other opportunity. This significant event can effect a quantum leap to a higher level of function for the children (the abstraction of the Katchina spirit as separate from the concrete vessel of the Katchina Dancer). A dramatic and painful event provides the impetus for further growth and development within a patient.

The children's understanding of the masked dancers is ritually transformed, which transforms the child, who then accepts the realness of Katchinas on another level. Their embodiment through the child's own relatives ultimately completes a circle and allows the child to eventually become a Katchina Dancer as well. The notion of a dance between two alternate states of reality is clear: there is a relationship between the Divine and the actions of real people. The adult sees both a Katchina and a human dancer at the same time. The child sees only a Katchina. The ceremony is a celebration of both.

SOUTH: INITIATION AND LEARNING

There is a traditional Twana story (Elmendorf, 1993) that comes from the Pacific Northwest about a boy who went camping on the wrong side of the tracks one night, and met Dashkaya. Now Dashkaya is a distant relative of *At'Atlilya,* the one the white people call Bigfoot or Sasquatch. She's not alone. She's got sisters. But we won't concern ourselves with her sisters right now.

This little boy had not actually gotten lost. He had left home that morning to go hunting and was enjoying the day so much—it was bright and sunny, one of those rare days in the Pacific Northwest—that he wandered too far from his home to make it back before sundown. So he thought, "I'd better just camp out where I am for the night and start back first thing in the morning," just as his elders had taught him to do. Well, it wasn't long before Dashkaya smelled the boy. She's got a supernatural sense of smell, and for a good reason. She eats children. As legend has it, she carries a big basket on her back that can hold as many children as she can eat in a sitting. And she's always hungry. This little boy had just gotten settled in when all of a sudden he heard an eerie whistling in the dark. After a while the clouds slowly moved across the face of the moon to reveal a giant, hairy figure standing quite still, looking directly at him. Now this boy had taken Monsters 101 and knew that what was standing over him was none other than Dashkaya, the celebrated devourer of children. Besides, nothing human could smell as bad as she did.

Now Dashkaya knew that if she were going to nab this morsel of a kid, she'd have to use cunning. She heard the boy's stomach grumbling from hunger. He hadn't caught much that day to eat. She put on the best face she could muster under the circumstances—and by this we mean she was so ugly, even a smile looked terrifying—and teetered over to the boy who was shaking rather uncontrollably.

"Know who I am?" she grumbled to the boy, who was now covering his eyes and nose. "Well, never mind what you've heard about me. I'm sure it's all negative. But it's all untrue. In fact—" she muttered, and leaned over to assess the boy's plump little arms, "—in fact," she continued saying, as she reached into the basket on her back, "I'm not really a bad person at all." She smiled, her teeth glinting in the slight light of the moon. "I know little children need lots of good food, and I bet you haven't eaten a thing all day." She stretched out her hand to the boy, and piled high on her palm were juicy berries. "Open your eyes," she screeched, despite herself. "I've got something good to eat here."

And he did, slowly at first, until he saw the hairy outstretched hand of Dashkaya, which resembled the hard claw of a bird of prey—an owl, perhaps. Piled high on her palm were the biggest, juiciest berries he had ever laid eyes on. Just then, they both heard his stomach grumble.

"Go on," Dashkaya purred with only a hint of impatience. After all, there were more children to catch and this one was taking forever to make up its mind. Well, there was no denying the boy was hungry. And children don't deny themselves things as adults might. Dashkaya knew that.

Often stories play with paradox: that what is true on one level of reality may be even truer on yet another level. The boy knows of Dashkaya. He knows, as a traditional audience knows, what happens when one accepts the offer of the berries. How many alcoholics and drug addicts accept the offer of the "first time" knowing what the possible consequences of their choice might be? How many times do people reach once again for the berries or alcohol or the drugs, thinking, "This time things will be different. This time it will be a different story"?

As the boy tentatively reached out his own hand, carefully avoiding the menacing talons, Dashkaya was busy wiping a sticky resin across her other palm, which she had carefully hidden behind her hairy back. And just as the moon was once again obscured by the clouds she struck out, smearing the boy across the eyes with that sap, blinding him. Grunting, she grabbed hold of him within his blanket with her talons and heaved the boy over her shoulder into her basket. "Now, maybe a little girl too," she thought to herself as she disappeared back into the woods, whistling her eerie song.

The traditional telling of the preceding story describes a routine hunting trip—something very ordinary that ultimately brings extraordinary consequences. The boy does exactly what he is told to do under the circumstances in which he finds himself. He camps out in the woods instead of attempting to make the long journey home by night. He makes a competent decision. Similar to the boy in the story, we too may make competent decisions based on our set of worldviews that might result in unexpected and unwanted consequences. The very act of making the best choices in one given circumstance might achieve the opposite of our intention.

This story teaches us that even when we do everything right, things can go seriously wrong. Everything we may have mastered in our lives up to this point, a successful career, family life, prestige among our peers—whatever the case may be—may not provide us with what we require to resolve or escape crisis in our personal lives when we meet the Dashkaya of alcohol or drug abuse, or any issue we may bring into therapy that we cannot seem to resolve. How many times have we made choices that led us into situations that seemed even more unmanageable than before? Perhaps, as the boy did, we think, "Since I'm hungry, I'll just eat those berries." The situation then escalates, and we find ourselves experiencing even greater challenges. The routines we enjoy in our lives, such as successful careers and happy family relationships, can be turned upside down by personal crisis in less than a moment's notice. We do not ask for these disruptions any more than the boy in the story wanted to meet Dashkaya. We may reach the point where anything we do based on the very best of intentions to extricate ourselves from something unpleasant seems to push us even deeper into Dashkaya's basket and apparently beyond our ability to solve the dilemma.

As the story goes, the boy is carried off to Dashkaya's campsite and dumped out of the basket onto the ground. Soon Dashkaya begins to build a huge campfire with which to barbecue the boy. She is so delighted at her catch that she begins to sing and dance around the campfire. The boy hears her song and his heart sinks, the same way that the moon has gone beyond the horizon. He begins to think about how his day started, wishing to himself that he had never walked so far from his home that morning. He wishes the day could start all over again. He begins to think about how the day began. It was warm and so wonderful. He remembers the warmth of the sun upon him, and as he does he draws closer and closer to the campfire to feel the heat against his face. The heat of the fire begins to warm the sap across his eyes. Ever so slowly, the sap begins to melt. Soon the boy can see out of one eye, and the world comes into focus.

He sees the hulking figure of Dashkaya dancing around the fire, and around him he sees many other children, blinded as he was, all around the campfire. Next to him is a little girl. He turns to her very slowly and tells her how he managed to melt the sap from his eyes. He tells her not to be afraid, that he has thought of a way of saving them all, and instructs the girl to turn to her neighbor and whisper the secret into her ear. Soon, all the children begin to see again. By now Dashkaya had been dancing for some time; her voice had grown hoarse and she was tired. After all, she was no young woman as far as supernatural monsters go. So she turned her back to the fire and faced the children she had readied for roasting. Just as she did, the children jumped up at once, ran directly toward her and pushed her with all their might into the fire. She began to burn; her long hair singed. She began to crackle and hiss and her burning body exploded into sparks which lit up the sky. From these points of lights emerged mosquitoes. That is why, even today, mosquitoes suck human blood.

WEST: REVELATION AND INSIGHT

When we work with psychospiritual models to understand the integration of myth with psychodynamic thought, we need a story along with the ability to draw a cognitive relationship to the story. Stories, whose richness operates on a metacognitive level of meaning, hold a cognitive "marker." We tell a story and then we ask, what is the moral of the story? In what way does this story relate to our own lives? The responses to the story encourage transformative experience.

It is interesting to note that in the Pacific Northwest, a wooden Dashkaya mask is sometimes carved to have two faces. On the surface, the mask is frightening to look at. It is constructed to represent the Dashkaya of legend (see Photo 5.1) with thick eyebrows, mouth exaggerated in an "O" shape, and long shaggy hair—unmistakably a monster to stay away from. Yet on the versions of these masks that are called "transformation masks," there is a string that operates a hidden shutterlike device. Once pulled, it opens the outside mask, splitting it in two, and another more human-looking mask is revealed (Napier, 1986).

The power of multiple layers of meaning is self-evident in its potential to transform. The mask represents two alternate levels simultaneously. Approaching this from a psychodynamic orientation, the mask in its duality represents the mechanism of projection. Underneath the monster exterior lies a more human face. The mask, insofar as it represents two simultaneous levels of reality, is a metacognitive construct. In the legend, Dashkaya doesn't die, but she is "transformed" into a cloud of mosquitoes. In much the same way, the goal of standard treatment moving through the primary and secondary axes along a diagnostic continuum is to restore the individual to the

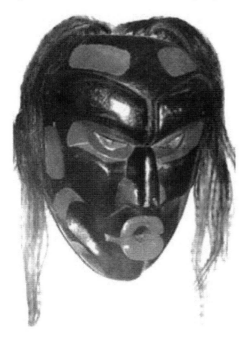

PHOTO 5.1. Native American Dashkaya Mask. Courtesy of Terry Tafoya.

most appropriate level of functioning. Clients may discover that the challenges they face in life may not disappear with awareness and their initiation into alternative ways of understanding. But the challenges may become manageable. It is important to note for the sake of clarification that there is the expectation of continued growth. For some therapists, for example, there is an expected continuum of guiding the client from psychosis to neurosis to a more "normal" standard of behavior. Just as Dashkaya transforms into mosquitoes, that particular story may end there, but there are other stories about Dashkaya. There are several points along the way where change is possible; we don't leave the client where we find him or her in our initial involvement.

In the Ai-yai-yesh Girl story, the heroine completes her medicine wheel. She begins her journey. She is initiated by the Cedar Tree to understand that there are other possibilities. Her eyes "open" in a new way and she learns to see in an alternative way, discovering the patterns that have always been around her. It is important to understand that the patterns were there all along, but she didn't know how to see them. The human dancers were always under the Katchina masks. The more-human mask hides beneath Dashkaya's monster mask.

The Ai-yai-yesh Girl manifests this learning in the construction of the baskets, and then brings the knowledge home to her community to integrate herself and this knowledge and to enrich those around her. Her journey, similar to the journeys of the audience, is not really over when the story ends. As long as breath is drawn, we continue to cycle through the medicine wheel over and over again—hopefully in an increasing spiral, so that each time we go through the four directions, we go through them at a higher level of development and understanding.

The boy did not plan to meet Dashkaya any more than a client might choose to face many of life's challenges: divorce, death, or any number of compelling unpleasant or pleasant circumstances. The story tells us that action is needed, but that it may be atypical or even counterintuitive. Unexpected resources, ones the boy did not stop to consider, appeared to him at the right time. Somehow, this boy realized that the fire which was meant to destroy him was also paradoxically the method of his survival, and ultimately the instrument of his own transformation. There is not the expectation that the client will make a quantum leap to wellness. Instead, there is the expectation of a series of small steps.

Working with the at-risk adolescent population presents many clinical challenges that mirror the journey of the young boy that meets Dashkaya. This Dashkaya story can be told to adolescents for it conveys to the listener a number of important moral concepts. (As noted earlier, stories often play with paradox and in so doing speak to many levels.) The therapist working from a Native American perspective can see the story acting out in a young person's challenges and behaviors. For many of the at-risk youth I (Nick) have worked with, Dashkaya was the specter of physical and sexual abuse and gang involvement.

A fifteen-year-old of Meso-American, Native, and Hispanic heritage with a history of drug and alcohol abuse, physical abuse by her father, and rape at the age of fourteen by her adult boyfriend (a gang member), was accepted into our six-month residential program. Heavily guarded and pseudomature, she responded to standard therapeutic technique with guarded suspicion and finally with open hostility. This client, a former gang member herself, felt anger, derision, and guilt toward her mother, whom she perceived as a weak woman who could not protect her from an abusive father. The deaths of many of her peers who were victims of gang violence had hardened this client's resolve to survive in a toxic environment that both terrified her and also gave her a strong sense of identity.

A very gifted artist, this female client spent much of her time drawing pictures of tough, physically powerful and intimidating women that appeared ready for battle. In many of these drawings, scars resembling barbed wire were drawn into the faces of her subjects, and a tear in one or both eyes.

Our sessions began to focus more and more on these drawings and on the intent of this artwork from the perspective of this client, who felt more and more a growing sense of helplessness, fear, and sadness as her figures grew more and more severe and angry. Similar to the boy who met Dashkaya and remembered the warmth of the sun, it took many months of building trust for this client to release years of pain, loss, and grief. What seemed most dangerous and therefore most counterintuitive to this fifteen year-old girl was the expression or demonstration of vulnerability, softness, or openness, traits that were perceived by this client to be signs of weakness. To remember a time—even if it was created in herself—that she felt safe and loved was a daunting task. The years of abuse had sapped her vision.

This client eventually gained insight into the choices she could make to explore empowerment on many levels, including gender roles within her culture of origin as well as the manner in which she could exercise her own competence and power. After five months of counseling, this client expressed an interest in speaking to other teens similar to herself who were involved in gangs and to use her artwork to express the violence of gang involvement. As was the case for the boy who met Dashkaya and informed and shared his vision with the other children, the transformative circle or hoop for this client was completed when she reentered her own community and moved into her mother's home in the inner city with a new set of eyes to see the world around her.

One Japanese proverb says, "Learning without wisdom is like a load of books on the back of an ass." It is vital to the survival of the community that those who are initiated return to let the community know what has been seen and learned. In the Dashkaya story, had the boy kept his "insight" to himself, he would have perished. By sharing his insight, he was able to increase his circle of support and bring about transformational change. His individual change allows institutional change. In the same manner the former Ai-yai-yesh Girl returns and changes forever her community through the creation and use of her baskets.

NORTH: TRANSFORMATION AND SYSTEMIC CHANGE

In a crisis situation, it is often after we reach a point of no return or hit bottom that we begin to consciously accept that the situation is well beyond our ability to control. We are metaphorically blinded for a time and thrown into the bag of a careening monster; very real and mounting danger exists and we may lose everything. We sadly conclude that escape is not possible in the same way through denial or indulging even more in the same behavior. What has worked in the past no longer works. It is important to focus on what remains, on our ability to grow and to transform beyond what has happened—even after so much has been temporarily lost: our freedom to make choices, our ability to act decisively, our power to fight Dashkaya. Despite this, what remains is hope for recovery.

One such case involved a female client in her thirties, half Native American and half white. She had been sexually abused by her non-Native father. She had been hospitalized with depression and had been suicidal. She was also at the point of exhaustion from a combination of work, raising a family, and attending seminary full-time to become a minister. At the suggestion of a mutual friend, she contacted me (Terry) and asked for my assistance. I spoke with her primary therapist, and decided to do a naming ceremony.

Names for Native American people usually have extreme significance. These are not the legal and standard names most people are familiar with, but rather names of a more traditional nature, most often in the language of the tribe. In some Native Nations, it is believed that upon death one will be called by the Creator by the Indian name and therefore to not have a true name means being spiritually lost. In many communities, names are inherited, where one is named after a deceased relative, or one may share a name with a living person. In other situations, a name may be created or dreamed by a ritual or elder (or in some communities, by a Two-Spirit person or someone from an alternative gender role).

Names are also frequently used as a focus for meditation and self-examination. In other words, when one is troubled, one's name can be called on in the sense of trying to see how the resources of one's name may influence a challenge or problem. For example, one of my names would translate as "Child of the Eagle." When faced with a challenge, I might think about how an eagle would see the situation—perhaps at a great distance, flying high, so that the problem doesn't seem to be so overwhelming but is put into perspective.

In this instance, I had decided to do the naming ceremony for a number of reasons. First of all, it allowed the patient to die symbolically—in terms of addressing her suicidal ideation and as a way of dealing with her incest abuse issues—and yet to be reborn as a new person, since the naming is seen as a type of spiritual rebirth. Given that the patient did not grow up in her own Native family (the mother had died when she was very young, and she was reared by her non-Native father), the Indian name would also confer a sense of status and recognition within the local Native community. Finally, it also permitted future pacing, for she was instructed that she would need to sponsor a giveaway within a year after receiving her new name. In accordance with tradition, she would have to give away gifts in one of the longhouses before her name could be announced formally in the community. Naming ceremonies will almost always involve a giveaway. This allowed her to focus on getting well enough to return to work in order to be able to pay for objects that would be given away in the ceremony, rather than place her focus on her depression.

Various hospital personnel were formally invited to the ceremony, along with her husband and other members of her family. The escorting is a very standard procedure for most naming ceremonies in the Pacific Northwest. For example, if a male is getting named, then two men will walk side by side with the namee. If it is a woman, then two women are chosen. Because of her mixed heritage, I requested that she be escorted into the naming by a Native friend of hers and also a non-Native (in this case, the clinical director of the program). After drumming and singing, the name was announced, the English translation of which would be Salmon Woman, meaning "She Who Is Renewed." The following story was then shared that explicated the name.

Long ago, a Woman of the Waters fell in love with a Native Man. She took him to meet her father, the Chief of their People. To honor the man he sponsored a feast and instructed all present that they must return to him all the heads, tails, skin, and the bones of the salmon they were about to eat. Being contrary by his nature, the man wondered why he must do this, and secreted a bone between his cheek and gum. When the salmon had been eaten, the Salmon Chief gathered the heads, tails, skin, and bones together and put them into a basket. He made as if to throw the remains into the water once, twice, thrice, and then on the fourth time threw them into the water. The water began to bubble and churn, and from the center stepped the Chief's youngest son, but he limped as he came forward.

"Who has kept out a bone?" questioned the Salmon Chief. "My son is not whole!" Quickly the man brought forth the missing bone and gave it to the Chief, who repeated the ritual.

This time the boy stepped forward without a limp, fully restored. The Salmon Chief told the man that because of the love his daughter had for him, the Salmon People and the Humans would enter into a covenant. As long as the Salmon were treated with respect and this ritual would be carried forth by the Humans, the Salmon would return to feed the people.

Just so, the First Salmon Ceremony remains a significant part of Northwest traditions. The first salmon of the season is caught and called by the Salish people, *see-yapi* which roughly translates as "noble one." The fish is escorted on a bed of fern and sung in (as the namee is brought in with drumming, rattles, and song). The salmon is cooked, and the head, tail, skin, and bones are saved, to be taken and thrown into the spawning grounds. This way the Circle of the Salmon is completed. The analogy of the salmon of Native tradition to the Christian Eucharist is well known in the Pacific Northwest. The story also plants the idea of renewal and rebirth, and links into the patient's self-image of someone who gives to her community but with the additional suggestion to not give away oneself completely, in the manner of Old Mother Hubbard of nursery rhyme fame.

The patient was released from the hospital the following day, and within the year she successfully had her giveaway in one of the longhouses, as scheduled. In an interesting side note, a few weeks afterward, she called me. She was having a series of disturbing dreams related to the incest that she felt was connected with her ongoing therapy, and she wanted to know if she needed to fully reexperience the traumatic emotions related to her past. On a personal and professional level, I don't think that is absolutely necessary, but I hesitated to tell her that since I was not her primary therapist, and I was unsure of her primary therapist's training and focus. The clinical director of the program was a mutual friend. She later telephoned me to say that the patient had gone into a trance state, apparently demonstrating the nonverbal signs that she had exhibited during the naming ceremony, and stated, "I don't have to have the dreams." She later reported that the dreams had stopped.

SELF-CARE AND INTEGRITY: GUIDES FOR THE HEALER

One of the additional Native American teachings is that every time you heal someone, you give a piece of yourself away, until at one point you will need healing yourself. In many of the Pacific Northwest communities, the "patient" is placed on a chair in the center of a circle of his or her family, friends, and supporters. The Indian doctor, a term much more frequently used than "medicine man" or "medicine woman," will often tell those present, "One day you will sit in the chair yourself." This serves as a reminder that those involved in healing must never think of themselves as superior to the patient, but that we are all part of a great circle and a circle has no "head" or "top." In fact, in some teachings, one is not permitted to work full-time as a healer until after retirement from a more standard occupation. This stems from the idea that if your income is derived from working only with "sick people," then you'll have an unconscious desire to keep them sick or your income would stop.

There is a very respected and beloved teacher, spiritual leader, and healer of the Twana people from the Skokomish Reservation: Bruce Miller, or Subiyax (his Indian name). Well known as a traditional storyteller, he was asked in the spring of 1999 to present at a multicounty coalition on mental health services for Native people on the many reservations located within the counties. After dinner, he was requested to tell some stories before children came in from the Port Gamble S'Kallam Reservation to perform their Coastal style dancing. He closed with the following story:

> Long ago, it was very important to seek out one's Power . . . what we call in our language your *skalulitut*. Bear had fasted and done all the proper things in seeking his Spirit Power, and returned successfully. He invited all the animal people to his

longhouse to provide them a feast in celebration of his vision quest. He worked hard, and he and his relatives provided all sorts of different and delicious foods the various people loved to eat: clams and salmon and sea urchin eggs, roots and berries. The people were very impressed by how much there was and how many different types of foods there were. There was only one thing missing. In the tradition of the Northwest Coast, people liked to dip their food in oil. This was considered very high class and chiefly people traded for the oil, and it was most normally seal oil or oil from oolikan or the candlefish. When the people started to complain about not having oil, Bear announced it was time to demonstrate his new Spirit Power. His relatives brought out bowls made of shells and placed them around the fire. The people all watched in anticipation.

Bear began to sing his new spirit song. "Hu hu yea, hu hu yea, hu hu yea hee ha, hu hu yea hee ha." As he held his hands over the bowls, oil began to drip out, and his relatives passed the oil among the people to use.

Bluejay was most impressed of all. When he left, he called all of his relatives together and told them, "Bear has done something very wonderful and has shown how truly high class he is with his Spirit Power. The truth is that we are not considered high class at all, is this not true?" Sadly, his relatives nodded their heads in agreement.

Now, it was well known that Bluejay was always curious about what others did and always tried to imitate them, which always brought him sorrow and pain. He never thought about how really hardworking the people he was trying to imitate had been and how much preparation their actions took. He just saw the results of the labor and always thought he could do it as easily as they made it look. So he turned to his relatives and said, "And as you know, I myself recently went on a vision quest. Do you remember a while back when I was gone for a few days?" The others looked at each other. No one could remember Bluejay having been gone. "Well, no matter. Anyway, I myself have received a Spirit Song, and I want us to gather food to provide a feast for people and then I will demonstrate my new song for everyone to admire and we will be proclaimed truly high class people."

His relatives worked very hard (much harder than Bluejay, who said he needed to rest to make sure his Spirit Power was at its full strength) gathering food to use in the feast, and invited the people to Bluejay's longhouse on the following full moon. The people were impressed by the variety of foods but again noticed that such a wonderful feast was spoiled by the absence of oil to use for dipping. When Bluejay heard them start to complain, he announced that he was now ready to demonstrate his new Spirit Song. His relatives put shell bowls around the fire and waited in eager anticipation. Soon they all would be recognized as coming from a high-class family. Bluejay stood up and stretched, trying to remember Bear's song. He hadn't really been paying that much attention to the song itself; he had been thinking of how wonderful it would be for the people to admire him singing it. He cleared his throat and sang, "Hu Hu yuh—hmmm—Yah Hu Hu Hu . . . " and as he held his hands (really they were his feet) over the fire, he tried so hard to remember the song that he didn't notice his feet were beginning to char and burn from the heat of the fire. His toes began to curl up.

Bear stood up and pulled Bluejay away from the fire, saying, "Look, my people—look what happens when you do not truly respect the *skalulitut*. A sacred song is never something that you can steal; it is not something you can pretend to have. And now Bluejay will be marked for life, for he will never be able to walk again. " And just so, today the Bluejay cannot walk like a normal bird, a bluejay can only hop. And if you look closely at his feet, you will see they are charcoal gray and curled up as if they had been burned in a fire.

The storyteller finished his story and rolled his wheelchair off the floor to make room for the young dancers entering. The previous year, he had been moving a desk filled with heavy drawers of books. "I thought, 'Well, I should really take the books out,' but then I said to myself, 'Nah, I'm a big macho man. I can just lift the whole thing up.' "

When he did, one of the drawers fell out on his foot. Because of his diabetic condition, he had no feeling in his feet, and he did not recognize the seriousness of his injury. His foot had actually been broken. By the time he sought treatment, three toes had to be amputated due to gangrene. He continued to have problems with the foot, which was eventually amputated as well. A friend from eastern Washington State was assisting him and spun him around too quickly in his wheelchair, hitting the newly stitched leg and ripping out the stitches.

He then acquired septic blood poisoning and was very close to death. The leg was eventually amputated a few inches below the knee. He has been adjusting very successfully to the loss of his leg through crutches and a wheelchair, joking about how difficult it was for him to use the clutch.

During traumatic events, Native people will use the stories they grew up with to make sense of their lives. A significant event such as the loss of a leg makes one question of, "Why did this happen to me? What is the meaning of this?" Bruce Miller also used the story in yet another way. As I pushed his wheelchair away, we passed the director of the agencies attending the conference. He went into great detail with the director of how we were related to each other, and that I had the hereditary right to use the stories and songs of his family, knowing that I would be presenting the following day. He was explaining to the director that my use of the Twana songs and stories were legitimate—that I was no Bluejay. Stories can provide so many layers of meaning. In the Twana language, for example, the phrase "He hops like a bluejay" means that someone is a thief.

CONCLUSION

In using Native American traditions and stories as part of the healing process it is important to be respectful not only to the *skalulitut* but to all beings. An elder stood before those assembled in the longhouse a few years ago and said, "When I was a girl, we were taught that everything was a person. The chair was a person. The dish was a person. The table was a person. We are all people; we are just different types of people. It is when we stop treating so-called 'objects' with respect that we also learn not to respect one another." Often well-meaning non-Native people will approach traditional spiritual people and elders wanting to learn from them but with no realization that the conventional educational methods they are most familiar with are not what they will find in Native communities. Learning how to do a ceremony or a ritual can take a tremendous amount of preparation and training, because it is clearly understood that the action itself is only a small part of the actual process (see Photo 5.2).

For example, a number of years ago, a group of Navajo people was given Super 8 video cameras and asked to record the process of mak-

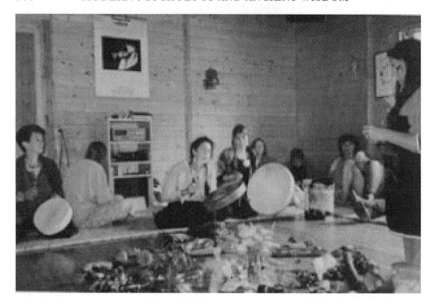

PHOTO 5.2. Workshop in Tuscany on Native American Ritual. Courtesy of Terry Tafoya.

ing rugs (the Navajo are well known for their weaving arts). When the thirty-minute films were returned and developed, they were very similar in content. They would show twenty-four to twenty-six minutes of sheep, of sky, of land, of water, of flowers, and only the last four to six minutes of the films would show someone actually weaving the rug itself. In other words, just as Zen archery teaches that the least important moment is the releasing of the arrow, so too do many Native peoples recognize that many actions are extremely complex and not easily understood.

In a relatively short period of time, a person might be taught how to make a basket; but that won't make the person a basketmaker, as the Aye-yai-yesh Girl was. That is why, historically, individuals wanting to learn to "be" would be apprenticed to someone who was already a master in the field of interest. If you wanted to become a basketmaker, you would actually live in the household of the master basketmaker. In this way, you could observe how a basketmaker responds to the world when he or she is not making baskets, which, of course, is the majority of his or her life. Thus, a basketmaker sees the world in a fundamentally different way than a hunter will, and the hunter sees the world in a different way than the healer will. Learning to see in this manner is not something you acquire from a six-week course in basketmaking that meets an hour a day.

Too often non-Natives try to observe a Native event or ritual, and like Bluejay, take away a part of it without fully understanding the implications of what they are doing. For example, in most Native traditions, a vision quest would never be attempted alone. It is understood that not all spirits are those with the best interests of human beings at heart. There are some very potentially dangerous things out there besides Dashkaya. A vision quest is fully understood by Native people as a potentially life-threatening event, and it is treated accordingly.

Some non-Natives seem to take the attitude, again, like Bluejay, that they see something done, figure out the "active ingredients," and leave out the bits and pieces that they don't see as being relevant. They lack the understanding that the "irrelevant" pieces are part of the whole and of the balance of things. This is the same attitude that causes lumber industries to see some trees as "desirable" for economic reasons and other trees as "waste" because they are not profitable, but being blind to what role the "waste" plants play in the total ecology.

Stories tell us that a difficult, painful experience—be it along the lines of addiction, physical or sexual abuse, or loss—has in it the dormant seeds and the potential for transformation. The Native philosophy holds that each transformation brings about the necessary teachings and experiences for the next crisis and transformation, and that this process is a circle of greater and greater self-awareness as well as awareness of one's place in the universal circle of friends, family, nation, and beyond.

So we tell the stories to let the insight be passed on in a way that allows people to remember who they are—to let them see the shadow without running away. We tell the stories to let people remember that there are always alternatives. We tell the stories and, sometimes, the stories tell us.

REFERENCES

Beck, P., Walters, A., and Francisco, N. (1977). *The Sacred: Ways of Knowledge, Sources of Life*. Tsaile, AZ: Navajo Community Press.

Elmendorf, W.W. (1993). *Twana Narratives: Native Historical Accounts of a Coast Salish Culture.* Seattle: University of Seattle Press.

Griffin, S. (1992). Author's personal notes from her keynote address at the Phenomenology Conference at the University of Wisconsin, LaCrosse.

Napier, D.A. (1986). *Masks, Transformation and Paradox.* Berkeley: University of California Press.

Neihardt, J.G. (1961). *Black Elk Speaks: Being the Lifestory of a Holy Man of the Oglala Sioux* (Trans.). Lincoln, NE: University of Nebraska Press (Originally published 1932. New York: William Morrow).

Tafoya, T. (1990). Circles and Cedar: Native Americans and Family Therapy. In Saba, G.W., Karrer, B.M., and Hardy, K.V. (Eds.), *Minorities and Family Therapy* (pp. 72-97). Binghamton, NY: The Haworth Press, Inc.

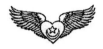

SUFISM

Sufism is a path of the heart leading to union with the Beloved. Native Middle Eastern and Sufi practices focus on helping students and clients to understand their inner reality, to find purpose in life, and to recognize diversity in their feelings and interior states. These healing processes also enable practitioners to discover healthy ways to relate to self and others. Stages of development are facilitated by movement, sound, breathing, body awareness, and depth work with the inner self *(naphsha)*. The focus of these practices is to experience love in all of its varieties of expression. This is more than a warm, "feel-good" experience that can be lost at a moment's notice; it is rather an incomparable union of hearts that goes beyond any romantic ideal or mental concept. This is the love that illuminated the Sufi poet Jelaluddin Rumi's heart, teachings, turning, and poetry.

> If you want what visible reality can give you,
> you're an employee.
> If you want the unseen world,
> you're not living your truth.
>
> Both wishes are foolish,
> but you'll be forgiven for forgetting
> That what you really want is
> love's confusing joy.

And gamble everything for love,
if you're a true human being.
If not, leave this gathering.
Half-heartedness doesn't reach into majesty.
You set out to find God,
but then you keep stopping for long periods
at mean spirited roadhouses. (Barks, 1993, p. 45)

Dr. Neil Douglas-Klotz explains how Sufi traditions use movement to increase awareness. As practitioners develop a more subtle awareness of movement they also develop a heightened awareness of transpersonal influences and energies. Aspects of the personality are illuminated and the potential for spiritual awareness is increased. This knowledge of body, movement, and breath is integrated in a modern-day manifestation of Sufism found in the Dances of Universal Peace, which are practiced worldwide. Dr. Douglas-Klotz explains how these dances facilitate community, encourage peace and healing, and awaken subtle awareness offering alchemical transformation. They are also used in groups for the developmentally disabled, in substance abuse recovery programs, and in special education settings.

This chapter encourages the reader to listen to the inner prompting of the heart. Human beings long for something more meaningful to guide them in this new millennium. In a world dominated by the Internet and other rapid-fire means of communication, Sufism conveys a message of healing that leads to the one true love that unites us all.

Chapter 6

The Key in the Dark:
Self and Soul Transformation
in the Sufi Tradition

Neil Douglas-Klotz

Once upon a time . . .

It is late at night. The legendary wise fool, Mulla Nasruddin, is crawling on his hands and knees under a corner streetlight. A close friend discovers him and, thinking that Mulla may be a little drunk, tries to help:

"Mulla, let me help you up! Do you need help to find your way home?"

"No . . . no, my friend. . . . I've lost the key to my house. Here . . . get down on your hands and knees and help me look."

Groaning, Mulla's friend lowers himself onto the hard pavement and begins to crawl around. He makes a thorough search, peering into all the crevices in the cobblestones, gradually and laboriously widening his search. After what seems like hours, his knees are aching. No luck.

"Mulla, I've looked everywhere within thirty feet. Are you sure you lost your keys here?"

"No . . . actually, I think I lost them about a block away, over there."

"Mulla, Mulla—you idiot! Why are we wasting our time here then?"

"Well, the light was better here . . ."

Sufism is a tradition of contrasts and paradoxes. To understand it, one must go beyond stereotypical images of turbans, long robes, and whirling dervishes. Although Western culture has taken Sufi poetry and teaching stories, like the previous one, to its heart, it tends to see them as entertainment, divorced from their original educational and therapeutic context. This is not wrong, because the stories and poetry convey truths that the subconscious mind recognizes, even if the conscious mind does not understand them. At the same time, Sufism presents a very profound psychology aimed at self-realization, which it defines as becoming a fully human being.

This chapter shows how psychospiritual theory and practice from the Sufi tradition can inform a person's psychological healing and soul journey. It begins with a necessary yet brief bit of history and background, then proceeds to examine, from a psychological standpoint, the best-known component of Sufism: Sufi stories and poetry. The middle part of the chapter discusses the view of the soul in the Sufi tradition as a multilayered, multifaceted reality, more akin to a community than an individual. Toward the last third of the chapter, I examine, from a psychological view, practical techniques used by Sufi teachers to accomplish these goals, including breathing, body awareness, sound, music, and movement, including dance and whirling. The chapter also contains several brief case studies. To conclude, I examine application of some of these practices to Western psychotherapy and other integrative health models.

HISTORY AND BACKGROUND

The term *sufism* simply means "wisdom" and was first given to a collection of mystical practices and training about 300 years after the time of the prophet Muhammad (peace and blessings upon him).

Sufis disagree about their origins. Some say that their practices go back to ancient Egypt or previous native mysticisms in the Middle East. Other Sufis say that Muhammad first brought a mystical-spiritual path (Sufism) which was later formulated into a religious organizational system that came to be identified with the word *Islam,* which simply means "surrender to divine Unity." In this view, Sufism is not the esoteric side of Islam (as most sources explain it); rather, the original was Sufism. For this reason, some Sufi groups in the Middle East and Asia as well as in the West allow practitioners of Judaism, Christianity, Hinduism, and other religions to become Sufi students.

Still other Sufis take a more narrow approach and view Sufism as a later mystical offshoot from Islamic religion, with the necessity that practitioners follow particular, culturally defined rules of worship and practice.

In relation to all this, it is simplest to say that Sufism represents a surviving form of Middle Eastern mysticism. The various Sufi orders and schools throughout the world differ in many respects but are united in their view of the soul, as well as in their emphasis on the need to practice remembrance (called *dhikr*) of divine Unity. Some Sufi schools use primarily silent meditation; others employ music and movement. Some use stories, poetry, or dream interpretation for transformations; others emphasize practical work in the world.

Rather than proceed in the abstract, the next section examines specific examples of Sufi stories and poetry in order to reveal some of the psychological underpinnings that unite all Sufi approaches. In the same way, a traditional Sufi teacher generally proceeds from concrete to abstract, from experience to concept.

THE ECOLOGY OF MIND
IN SUFI STORIES AND POETRY

Traditionally, Sufi stories are not artistic performances. Instead they arise within a spiritual community where the mutual search for wisdom demands a response to the moment, not a rehearsed enactment. The stories are often interspersed with spiritual practices or meditations that prepare the way for them or that lead one to the doorway of an experience the story implies.

Sufi stories may express humorous, sad, or mixed emotions, but generally they are not moralistic, nor is there one particular point to "get," as in a joke or riddle. The stories may have many layers; the most obvious ones often give way to the more subtle only with time and experience.

For instance, the story of Mulla Nasruddin that begins this chapter may seem utterly absurd. Yet upon reflection, how often do we look for answers to problems in ways that we are used to looking, even if they are not effective? The Western Sufi Ahmed Murad Chishti (Murshid Samuel L. Lewis, d. 1971) once said, "The reason we don't solve problems is that the answers interfere with our concepts" (Cohn, 1972). We tend to look with and through our conscious mind, rather than going into the shadow side of our subconscious where the answers may lie. On another level, we can see all of the characters and elements of the story as occurring within one psyche: Mulla, the friend, the light, the street corner, and the key.

In general, most Sufi stories aim to help us "unlearn," that is, to go beyond the emotional boundaries and mental concepts that enclose the sense of who we think we are. As we go beyond these boundaries, we find ourselves in the province of what one may call "wild mind." We discover an inner landscape that is both richer and less controlled than the safety of fixed ideas and rules. Gregory Bateson (cited in Donaldson, 1991) called this type of approach "ecology of mind," recognizing that consciousness operates much more like an ecosystem than anything else, and that "mind" is embedded in an ecological reality, within and without.

Seven hundred years earlier, the Persian Sufi Mevlana Jelaluddin Rumi said something similar (Barks translation, 1990, p. 113):

> The inner being of a human being
> is a jungle. Sometimes wolves dominate,
> sometimes wild hogs. Be wary when you breathe!
>
> At one moment gentle, generous qualities,
> like Joseph's pass from one nature to another.
> The next moment vicious qualities
> move in hidden ways.
>
> A bear begins to dance.
> A goat kneels!

As we recover a sense of the wild within, we may also come into a new relationship with nature outside of us. Each being in the natural world is beautiful and of value in itself: each is a unique face of the inexpressible Only Being, the divine Beloved.

Specific aspects of Sufi spiritual practice work with the part of our psyche *(nafs)* called the "animal soul" and even the "plant soul." The arrogance of considering only humanity worthy of an interior life is renounced. One begins to realize that no adequate life of any kind—"spiritual" or "practical"—is possible without considering the whole of our nature, that which we fear as well as enjoy. A predecessor of Rumi, the thirteenth-century Persian Sufi Mahmud Shabistari says in his *The Secret Rose Garden* (Douglas-Klotz, 1995, pp. 114, 132):

Look around you!

This world is tremendously mingled:
Angels, devils, Satan, Michael—
all mixed up like seed and fruit!
Atheist with fundamentalist,
materialist with mystic.

All cycles and seasons,
years, months, and days
converge at the dot of now:
"In the beginning" is "world without end."

This holistic or integrative point of view was also present from the beginnings of Islamic science (a science that did much to help Europe out of its own Dark Ages through the Moorish influence in Spain). As the Sufi scholar Seyyed Hossein Nasr (1968, pp. 3, 5) notes in *Man and Nature,* written more than thirty years ago:

> For a humanity turned towards outwardness by the very processes of modernization, it is not so easy to see that the blight wrought upon the environment is in reality, an externalization of the destitution of the inner state of the soul of that humanity whose actions are responsible for the ecological crisis. . . .
> [Some Western] thinkers forget that the pure monotheism of Islam which belongs to the same Abrahamic tradition as Judaism and Christianity never lost sight of the sacred quality of nature as asserted by the Quran, and that Oriental Christianity and Judaism never developed the attitude of simple domination and plunder of nature that developed later in the history of the West.

In this sense, Sufi stories and poetry represent an early ecopsychology; this is no doubt the reason why they appeal to the modern Western mind, which has lived for hundreds of years in a cosmology that divides humanity from nature and the divine. One of the main insights of ecopsychology says that much of what we call a personal psychological problem finds its roots in a deep collective denial and despair about what is going on in the natural environment.

In many Sufi stories, we find that our relationship to animals and nature is not only symbolic of our inner state but that we humans can become reflected in the inner lives of animals. To continue the section from Mevlana Rumi (Barks translation, 1990, p. 113):

> Human consciousness goes into a dog,
> and that dog becomes a shepherd,
> or a hunter.

> At every moment a new species rises in the chest—
> now a demon, now an angel, now a wild animal.

> There are also those in this amazing jungle
> who can absorb you into their own surrender.

> If you have to stalk and steal something,
> steal from them!

In Sufi stories, the world of animals and nature is inexhaustibly wild and mysterious. According to a Sufi, our human efforts to "domesticate" nature parallel our attempts to domesticate and deaden our inner life by holding onto the past or projecting ourselves into the future through what Rumi calls elsewhere "imitation." A modern synonym for this word might be "addiction"—a mindless, unfeeling, repetitive action that distracts us from the present moment.

Only when the universe breaks through to shock us—through the death of someone close, falling in love, intense joy, or a confrontation with some experience we cannot categorize—do we wake from sleep. Again, from a different section of Mevlana Rumi's *Mathnawi* (Barks translation, 1991, pp. 16-17):

> A farmer once tied his ox in the stable.
> A lion came and ate the ox
> and lay down in its place!

> The farmer went out late at night
> to check on the ox. He felt in the corner
> and rubbed his hand along the flank of the lion,
> up the back, feeling the shoulder, and around
> the chest to the other shoulder.

The lion thinks, "If a light were lit
and this man could suddenly see,
he would die of the discovery.

He's stroking me so familiarly,
because he thinks I'm his ox."

So the imitator doesn't realize
what he's fooling with. God thinks,
"You fake. Sinai crumbled and split
with jets of blood streaming from it
for the sake of the name
that you say so thoughtlessly.

You learned it from your mother and father,
not from your own experience."

Metaphorically speaking, if all "lions" become our tamed oxen, either inner or outer, who will awaken us and how will the cycle of interdependence continue? Hearing poetry and stories such as this speaks in a deeper way to the psyche of the listener. They affirm a reality of wholeness that one may recognize only in dream, in the moments between sleeping and waking, while making love, or while fully engaged in play or artistic creation.

VIEWS OF THE SELF AND SOUL

The Sufi teacher works first with story, metaphor, poetry, spiritual practice, or music to get beyond and behind the blocks that the conscious mind puts up to avoid recognizing its greater (and often terrifying) place in the universe. Then, shifting points of view, he or she may step back from these teaching modes, and give the conscious mind a schema, map, or philosophy to help reorient it in harmony with the subconscious learning that has already occurred.

Behind the seemingly "wild" expression in Sufi story and poetry, we find a detailed and subtle view of the psyche. A teacher usually gives these maps to students only at a later stage, however, because the conscious mind too easily assimilates a map and mistakes it for the territory itself. For this reason, grand psychological "theories of everything" seem to the Sufi doomed to failure because they either trivialize a profound reality that cannot fully be made conscious or else fabricate another orthodoxy that becomes a philosophical dogma.

The psychology of Sufism centers on the subconscious self *(nafs)* and its present and potentially more conscious relationship with divine Unity (Allah) as soul *(ruh)*. This involves what the twentieth-century Sufi Hazrat Inayat Khan (d. 1927) called "the annihilation of the false ego in the real" (1960, p. 21). The *nafs* participates in the divine being in the same way that an individual quality of Unity (called *sifat*) participates in divine Essence (called *dhat*). Together divine Unity (Allah) and Essence *(dhat)* make up a psychologically male-female concept of the Sacred. Similarly, the individual soul can be said to have both male and female aspects that make up full humanity.

As mentioned in the section on stories and poetry, the *nafs* itself presents the many different faces of an inner ecology, including human and nonhuman potentials. In classical Sufi literature, various names for these potentials are given. I have provided English equivalents:

- The "animal/plant soul" presents an instinctual relationship with the natural world or cosmos.
- The "reciprocal, causally oriented soul" presents the give-and-take relationship of being human.
- The "harmonious soul" presents a relationship that is surrendered to the universal sense of purpose pervading the cosmos. This might manifest as an interior saintly life.
- The "blessing soul" presents a relationship that actively gives help in the form of what Sufis call blessing-magnetism *(baraka)*.
- The "knowing soul" presents an illuminated and illuminating relationship to its surroundings in which teaching (either verbally or nonverbally) may be present.

Once a student begins to realize, through spiritual practice, the many elements of the inner personality as well as the transpersonal dimensions of soul (which one initially feels as "beyond the self"), he or she may begin to feel overwhelmed. For instance, as a result of doing sacred movement practice in Sufism, more than one person has told the author, "I feel there's so much going on, I don't know what to do with it all!" At one moment, students will begin to feel all that's holding them back, inhibiting not only movement but all areas of life. At another moment, they may feel a very grand sense of the transpersonal, of the whole—of moving in union with another person, the group, or the divine Beloved.

Between these two extremes—personal limitation and boundless Unity—lie all the movement and personality training that needs to be done. As one narrows the gulf between personal limitation and divine freedom, one perfects one's movement, so to speak, in all areas of life. Form is an expression of quality of feeling in the eye of the teacher. As mentioned, the *nafs* does not respond well to concepts or verbal direction; it does respond to pictures, music, and body awareness sensations created through movement and dance. A teacher can tell much about students by watching their movements, for the body reflects and holds subconscious impressions and patterns—some helpful, some not.

Both classical and modern teachers of Sufism have regarded the *nafs* as proceeding through various gradations of refinement. These also relate to the refinement of breathing and its responsiveness as felt and shown in the body-mind, or *soma* (Suhrawardi, 1979, 127ff.; Khan, 1960, 166ff.).

For instance, the first phase of *nafs* may begin with the soma feeling nothing but its own outward sensations. The soma does not distinguish inward states or acknowledge feelings; it holds tension and rigidity in absolute and habitual patterns. Psychologically, the conscious self is totally driven by subconscious desires and impressions.

In the following phases, the soma begins to reflect more and more flexibility, until one reaches a stage in which feeling, thought, and movement are united. Limitations still exist, but one begins to be aware of the role that personality limitations play within a unified view of the whole being, that is, of the divine Essence *(dhat)* and Qualities *(sifat)*. At this level of self-acceptance, an individual becomes both a comfort and help to those around him or her. The person who has awakened the "blessing soul" *(nafs-i-salima)* becomes devoted to service and to delivering all others from the tyranny of "egoself," realizing at the same time that all beings are both inside and outside of the self. The modern Sufi Hazrat Inayat Khan commented on this: "There is one Truth, the true knowledge of our being, within and without, which is the essence of all wisdom" (Khan, 1960, p. 20).

Using any sort of hierarchical gradation encourages the tendency to rate one's progress and to become so preoccupied with it that one cannot move forward. This is why a sense of feeling, devotion, and compassion for others is cultivated at the outset. Students also continually need to apply it to themselves, as well as to realize that one actually goes through "stages of *nafs*" every day or even every moment. Nothing is lost. The inner ecosystem is simply known more fully. The development resembles an ascending spiral more than a ladder.

Consequently, a Sufi would say that a person's movement becomes more "spiritual" as it shows less domination by ego ("what others may think") and more integration with all levels of self—including body and emotions.

Because beginning students may find it most difficult to face their "inner demons," the Sufi teacher may initially attempt to direct their love and compassion to the transpersonal, the divine Beloved. Here also classical Sufism distinguishes gradations of surrender or effacement *(fana)* in the divine:

- *fana-fi-sheikh:* effacement in the personal teacher or guide
- *fana-fi-pir:* effacement in a teacher who has passed on
- *fana-fi-rasul:* effacement in a divine messenger, prophet, or human ideal
- *fana-fi-lillah:* effacement in the being of the One Being
- *fana-i-baka:* effacement in a resurrection into one's true nature

To give an example of the way this works in practice, the American Sufi Ahmed Murad Chishti (Murshid Samuel L. Lewis) revived a Sufi science of walking meditation or attunement. In one such practice, the student is encouraged to walk in the footsteps of one's teacher or imagine the rhythmic presence of the teacher as one moves (a practice called *tassawuri* or, literally, imagination) (Lewis, 1991).

When the student can easily move in effacement with one person, then that same sense of *fana* may be directed to a teacher, or the teacher's teacher, then to a human ideal (such as a saint or prophet), then ultimately to the Only Being. In the final stage of the process of *fana* one is effaced in one's own personality as it resides in total connection with the divine. This is a state expressed well by the medieval Christian mystic Meister Eckhart: "I see now that the eyes through which I see God are the eyes through which God sees me" (Fox, 1983, p. 21).

Because of this multilayered progressive approach to transformation, the teacher/student relationship takes on great significance. By definition, the student is intended to move beyond the teacher, who is primarily seen as a companion on the path. The relationship is so important that it is universally viewed in Sufism as being empowered by a living chain of transmission *(silsila)* that includes all past teachers of one's lineage.

According to Samuel L. Lewis (1986, p. 322), the "teacher" is the positive pole and the "student" the negative pole of one battery, which, strictly speaking, is empowered by the only Teacher (Allah). When current flows through the battery, due to the trust between both parties, then transformation occurs in both persons. In this regard, Hazrat Inayat Khan deals with Western psychological notions of projection and transference as an aspect of the mental/emotional world called the "palace of mirrors."

In all cases, it is the teacher's responsibility to stay as clear as possible, using his or her own therapeutic process or spiritual practice to make sense of what is going on. Teacher/student relationships in Sufism, as they have entered modern Western culture, have not been immune to confusion. For instance, certain traditional Sufi ways of relating respectfully, called *adab,* were linked to an underlying understanding of relatedness to one's community.

These ways were taken for granted in Middle Eastern or Eastern cultures, but are entirely unknown in Western culture, which sets a high value on individuality. Because of this, students of Sufism in the West may not understand the type of *adab* necessary for spiritual development, especially where the actual relationship may become shrouded in trappings from another culture. At the same time, teachers from the East, not understanding Western culture, have misunderstood the responses of their students.

In this regard, Sufism in the West has responded to the example of most professional associations of psychotherapists that have developed codes of ethics and models of peer supervision to help provide a "reality check" for therapists in these difficult areas of projection and counterprojection, which usually involve issues of money, touch, sexual behavior, and power. Similarly, several Western Sufi groups have set out ethical guidelines to properly inform both students and teachers.

To summarize, the Sufi teacher works with practices that empower transformation intensively (through the grades of *nafs*) and extensively (through the relationships of *fana*). Each stage of development—*nafs* or *fana*—may take years—or may happen in an instant. These developments approach the same point from two different angles. One starts with the personality; the other with the trans-personality; both move toward a unified holistic view of life where actions, thoughts, and feelings are harmonized. The Sufis call what harmonizes the diversity and paradox within and without by the simple name, heart *(qalb)*.

As one begins to experience and move with heart, a world of sensations is discovered within that one may not have been allowing oneself to experience. We are back in Rumi's "jungle" again.

Without this background, it is impossible to properly regard Sufi spiritual practices involving movement, walking meditation, and dance. To simply imitate certain whirling and circular movements in sacred dance performances without pursuing corresponding training in awareness and heart awakening does nothing but introduce novelty and nervous energy into the psyche. Ritual dance and movement in Sufism do not begin with large expressions but with the smallest nuances of body awareness. The following section summarizes the major areas of work in these practices.

PRACTICES: BREATH, SOUND, WALKING MEDITATION, DANCE, TURNING, AND REMEMBRANCE

Breathing

Sufi teachers often direct their students to experience the awareness of breathing as a link between where they feel limitation *(nafs)* and where they feel freedom *(fana)*. When one feels one's breathing centered in the heart, this sensation begins to represent the still point, the place of silence within the conflicting demands one begins to feel. Awareness of breathing in all its subtlety brings one an increasingly refined sense of body awareness similar to that cultivated by eutony, Feldenkrais, and other somatic arts therapies. The student progresses from simple awareness of the breath while walking, through awareness of the nuances of breath (its direction, duration, and intensity), to a gradual release of the blocks to breathing that inhibit movement and a fully human connection to life.

Breathing practices in the Sufi tradition both elicit greater awareness as well as interrupt habitual patterns that keep one separate from the breath of nature. In the use of these practices, one needs a teacher to ensure that one's habitual neurotic patterns of breathing are not displaced onto the practice—thereby making the practice itself part of the problem. In the "dance of the breath," as well as the following movement practices, one aims to elicit altered states of awareness, which students then discover as elements of their natural awareness that they have enclosed or limited. The practices do not normally aim to produce "trance" (in the commonly understood sense); they strive for greater awareness of the interconnectedness among the divine, humanity, and nature. In fact, in such states of awareness the separate naming of these three becomes pointless.

For instance, in a group somatic therapy conducted by the author, using Sufi breaths to the four elements (earth, water, fire, air) and their corresponding body awareness elements, participants reported the following insights and experiences:

Bones (earth): J wondered whether the earth could support her weight: could it stand it if everyone gave their weight? She had a "feeling of relief that I don't have to bear it all myself." Others breathed a sigh with that. F felt a sense of relief and comfort. C, and some others, noted where they were not willing to meet the earth or where they felt unable to give their weight. For people interested in spiritual things, this sensation often brings up resistance or a great sense of relief as real grounding is felt for perhaps the first time.

Muscles (water): B began to feel how he was using muscle as bone—to ward off attack. As he began to sense his muscles, he noticed where the fluidity had been stopped—the flexibility. As an administrator, this was a big issue with him. D said he noticed that he wanted to be both flexible and solid at the same time and sort out muscle from bone sensation. J pointed to her chest and said she felt muscles loosening there and a clearer relation of bone to muscle. She said this felt like letting water into the earth, that they could work together for her.

Blood (fire): JM said she felt she had to start with big movements to feel her blood, then gradually found her way to small ones, the beginnings of it. R had a hard time feeling this and stood still most of the time. D said he lay down and felt his heart pulsing but moving would have been too much. C said an image came up that temporarily blocked her way to the sensation: a large black horse with nostrils red and flaring and the face of a frightened woman nearby.

Skin (air): J said she had a hard time feeling her skin, but then bent over into a ball like a balloon and rose up quickly. She said she felt light-headed. R said he felt light everywhere but his head; it was still a solid mass, not skin. C recalled a sense of both lightness and relief; she can "go off" easily, she feels.

I encouraged the group to experiment with these awarenesses over the course of the day as they walked or talked with others. Which felt most comfortable? Which sensations did they often feel? These and similar explorations deepened over the course of eight sessions and developed into a type of movement awareness and therapy, similar to somatic disciplines such as eutony and Feldenkrais.

Sound and Body Resonance

As the breath becomes more perceptible and sensitive, one also becomes aware of the sensations in the body that occur as the breath becomes audible. Again, Sufis place specific emphasis on feeling sound in the heart area to integrate the feelings of above/below, known/unknown, light/dark. They believe that the resonance of certain phrases and words actually impels increasingly greater awareness of self and the divine. The Sufi science of *wazifa* (chanted phrases, including the ninety-nine sacred "names" of Allah, the *sifat-i-Allah*) aims at engaging and awakening the sense of feeling to small movements in the body that reveal both self and the divine within. These chants invoke qualities such as mercy, compassion, and forgiveness that can be awakened within an individual. The chants also include what Western psychology might call "shadow" qualities—shame, misdirection, confusion—to communicate with and acknowledge the whole range of feeling experienced by the *nafs*. According to one Sufi point of view, one misuses sound and chanting when these practices cause practitioners to enter trance states in which they become less aware of themselves as whole human beings.

The following is from a written case report of a client who used Sufi sound techniques to explore the relationship between his voice and the ability to express and feel emotion, as well as with issues of creativity:

> When I began, I had a very weak voice although with some melodic quality. I did not feel at all in touch with my body.
>
> Through the use of the various sound practices, I occasionally developed a vague sense of being enlivened and having more energy, but this sensation came and went. About one year after beginning, in a group musical practice, I experienced feeling as though sound were coming not from my vocal box, but from a place in the middle of my chest, near the pulmonary center. At the same time, I heard a ringing sound above the musical notes. These, I later found, were called overtones. I also felt a warm, expanding feeling from the heart and a kind of emotional release of joy.
>
> This condition came and went for another six months. Then I had another "heart-opening" experience, which was felt as both massive pain and release of tension around the heart; I cried uncontrollably and felt I was coming apart.
>
> Following this, I began to use the primary sound/music practice of finding a note that resonated in the heart, and singing that note every day for fifteen to twenty minutes, using various mantric sounds. At the end of about eight months, I could always find my way to this sound. At the same time, any catches in my throat, voice, or breath that came up I began to reexperience as inhibitions and old memories that prevented me from intoning a natural sound (that is, saying who I was).

Walking Meditation

At the same time that he initiated the Dances of Universal Peace (1965), Murshid Samuel Lewis introduced modifications and refinements of traditional Sufi walking practices, which encouraged the ability to distinguish various states of awareness and control them. Because walking is a movement used in everyday life, the walking meditations in this Sufi tradition further encourage bridging the gap between the seemingly divine and seemingly commonplace. Teacher training in the Dances of Universal Peace always includes training in walking meditation.

One source of these meditations is a traditional aphorism of the Naqshibandi Sufi order: "Look down and see whose feet are those that walk." (One might compare this with the use of walking meditation during a Zen Buddhist retreat.) In the introductory walking practices, the participant may be told simply to walk breathing "in the feet" or another part of the body, or to be aware of the rhythm of the breath. After becoming aware, one is enjoined to try a different rhythm by comparison, a different direction or intensity of breathing, or a different intention of feeling (for instance, walking toward a goal). One is asked to become aware of any changes in the inner state, and any thoughts or emotions that may arise.

The next step in refinement of the walking meditations involves concentration on breathing in different centers of the body or in attunement to the classical elements (earth, water, fire, and air). This involves altering the direction, intensity, and duration of the breathing and enlarging the body awareness to notice small differences of perception. For instance, students may be encouraged to feel the elements as the body awareness of the bones/ligaments (earth), muscles/connective tissue (water), heart/lungs/bloodstream (fire), and skin (air). These somatic correspondences were adapted by Hazrat Inayat Khan (1962) from traditional Sufi psychology. Research by the author has confirmed their usefulness in various therapeutic settings including substance abuse education. For instance, a heightened awareness of relaxed muscle/connective tissue while moving seems to mimic the somatic effects of alcohol in some cases (Douglas-Klotz, 1984).

Advanced practice in walking meditation uses rhythms associated with the alchemical planets in combinations with elements. Further walking attunement practices encourage the experiences of *fana* by walking in a breath-movement connection with another person. All of these variations aim at releasing the natural breath and movement available to the participant, so that the devotion elicited by the dance and other practices is available in a useful way throughout life.

The following excerpt is from a case study report of a group using Sufi walking practices to explore the experience of walking in the city of San Francisco. The therapeutic issues quickly surface in relation to the experience of both sound and breathing while walking:

We now proceeded another block downhill to the beginning of the financial district. The noise and activity increased. We crossed the street and went up to the large level plaza outside the Bank of America building. Some group members commented on the increased noise there. I asked them whether they could hear the sound of their own footfalls, even with all the noise. Or could they perhaps allow the vibration of their steps to come up through them all the way to the top? Was there any sense of their unique sound amidst the other noise?

The group members walked off in all directions around the plaza exploring their own sound. In about five minutes we came together again. J said that she felt her steps soften in order to hear them better. Paradoxically, she said, she needed not to press or tromp down so much in order to feel/hear the vibration through her. D said that she became aware of a vibration coming up from her feet all the way up the backbone and out the top of the head, giving her a completely new sense of alignment. Her eyes were sparkling.

E felt that it was very difficult to sense her own sound, but it was there if she listened closely. She said that she usually wore wooden clogs. This made the sound of her footsteps very loud and caused people to look at her as she approached. Wearing running shoes, she became aware of how she could listen for and feel the same vibration on a more subtle level. She felt this was a different way of making contact.

Dance

As one becomes aware of the movements within caused by breathing and sound, the prayers and sacred phrases so intoned or sung naturally cause one to begin to move the whole body in rhythm. As mentioned, this unity of intention and action is common to sacred dance in most native traditions. In the underlying native Middle Eastern tradition, one can see the expression of this principle in the story of David dancing before the altar of the Lord (2 Samuel 6:14, *The Holy Bible,* King James Version) in the Hebrew scriptures as well as in the tradition of Jesus dancing with his disciples on the evening before his crucifixion in the gnostic Acts of John (Elliot, 1996, pp. 60-62). In the aspect of this tradition that survives in Sufism, one can categorize various types of movements and their effects.

Strictly speaking, the term "Sufi dancing" is a misnomer. The dances most often referred to were originally named the Dances of Universal Peace (see Photo 6.1), and were first developed as a public form of sacred movement by the aforementioned American Sufi Ahmed Murad Chishti (Murshid Samuel L. Lewis, 1896-1971). Lewis was initially schooled and authorized as a teacher in a branch of the Chishti Sufi order, which was brought to Europe and the United States from India in 1910 by the Sufi Pir Hazrat Inayat Khan. Lewis himself also studied in India, Pakistan, and Egypt with a number of Sufi orders including the Naqshibandi, Suhrawardi, Qadri, and Rufai. The Dances of Universal Peace use movements derived from the practices of these orders as well as from a synthesis of spiritual dance techniques Lewis derived from his study with American sacred dance pioneer Ruth St. Denis (Lewis, 1986; St. Denis, 1996).

Toward the end of his life, Lewis began to develop this form of circle dancing with awareness of breath, sound, and movement, which he felt could be presented to the public as a means to expand one's sense of the self through devotion as well as to promote peace through

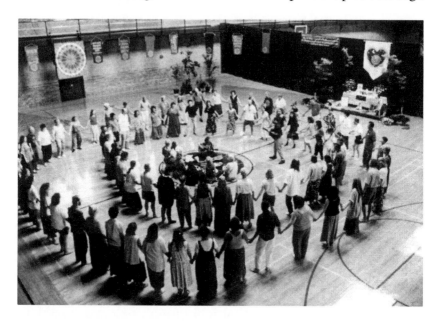

PHOTO 6.1. Dances of Universal Peace Gathering. Courtesy of Jon Harrison and the International Network for the Dances of Universal Peace.

the arts. In the later capacity, the Dances of Universal Peace use sacred phrases from most of the world's spiritual traditions, and participants are encouraged to feel the traditions uniting within themselves—in peace rather than at war. Variations of dances using folk-style partner movements encourage dancers to bring this experience into relationships with what the ego-self habitually sees as "others." Because this form of dance was done publicly, forms of imitation without feeling or training proliferated under the general rubric "Sufi dancing," and the term has sometimes come to mean any form of circle dance with singing.

Even such a public form of Sufi movement as the Dances of Universal Peace demands training if pursued over a period of time. Continued refinement of breathing and work with the personality are necessary. Proper teaching of each dance directs participants back to the feeling of the breathing and to the source of thoughts and emotions within. Devotion must be transmuted from a dualistic experience to one in which the subconscious *(nafs)* is encouraged to develop in the atmosphere of acceptance, expansion, and freedom that the dance creates. In this regard, specific applications of these dances have been made for therapeutic use with various populations (for instance, developmentally disabled, substance abuse groups, as well as in special education settings). The primary use of the Dances of Universal Peace remains that of an accessible form of devotional group dance in which the gap between participant and performer does not exist. From a psychological viewpoint, they combine movement reeducation, transpersonal therapy, and community building in a unified form that transcends these names.

Whirling and the **Sema**

Most of the walking meditations developed by Murshid Samuel Lewis also have a counterpart turning practice. The act of turning or whirling with a certain concentration helps focus one's breathing and body awareness. During turning, one can no longer visually spot without becoming dizzy, so attention is drawn to the center or element upon which one focuses. One develops through this practice an independent center of balance that can lead to a sense of "being turned" rather than turning. As one proceeds further, this experience of "not-self" is again revealed to have a home within.

The Turkish Mevlevi order of Sufis also uses turning in a formalized ritual that has been exquisitely developed over the course of 600 years to commemorate the passing of the founding *pir* of the order, Mevlana Jelaluddin Rumi. It was said that Rumi, upon learning of the death of his close friend and teacher, grabbed a pole in the marketplace and began to turn in both grief and ecstasy. Thereafter he began to express the pinnacle of Persian mystical poetry in his writings.

In this formal turning, or *sema,* one's attention must absolutely remain on the breath with a subvocalized form of *dhikr.* With arms upraised, one palm reaches up, the other down as the turning *semazen* presents the image of a funnel receiving from the heavens and giving to the earth. In his or her internal prayer, the *semazen* wishes to receive from the ultimate idealized divine and to bring this awareness fully into the body. The extensive training involved usually tests the subconscious *nafs* to the limit, but the beauty of the movement and music helps win its cooperation. As with other forms of Sufi movement, the so-called physical form of the Mevlevi turn is merely the doorway for exploring and reevaluating one's beliefs, impressions, and feelings about the self and God, as one goes through stages of *nafs* and *fana.* Although this is the most "choreographed" of Sufi movement practices, its choreography is designed for inner effect first rather than its impression on the observer (Friedlander, 1975).

Dhikr *(Remembrance)*

Dhikr is a traditional form of chanting and movement practice used by most Sufi orders. Participants usually sing or chant some form of the Arabic phrase *La illaha illa 'llahu* ("There is no god but God" or "There is no reality but Oneness"), or portions thereof, as a means of impressing the self with its origin and goal. *Dhikr* is performed in a variety of ways: seated, standing, moving in a circle or lines, and more or less vigorously depending on the Sufi order and the inspiration of the person leading the practice. The author experienced one *dhikr* practice with a Naqshibandi order in Lahore, Pakistan, in which the seated chant was accompanied by the counting of a sack of coffee beans.

Most orders reserve *dhikr* for initiates—those who have committed to a path of transformation through Sufism—although with more Sufi orders now establishing branches in the West the practice is sometimes done publicly. Nevertheless, there are good reasons to be conservative in this regard. Because *dhikr* does not focus on qualities (as does *sifat*) but on the essence of unity, it may be not be initially understood or assimilated by the subconscious and there may be more energy evoked than the body can assimilate without preparation.

In the currently male-dominated societies of the Middle East, this practice is often limited to men, and its evolution in this context has focused on the need to break down certain habitually male somatic rigidities (for instance, around the solar plexus). In more pluralistic societies, forms of *dhikr* have evolved that use a variety of movements appropriate to both men and women. There have traditionally been women Sufi teachers throughout Sufism's recorded history, although not in all orders or cultures (Cornell, 1999). Some researchers believe that this inclusiveness survives from earlier times in the desert mystical orders of the Middle East in which the aspect of God worshiped was typified female rather than male (Walker, 1983, p. 961).

TWENTY-FIRST-CENTURY APPLICATIONS

Although the more overtly ritualistic elements of Sufi practice may seem difficult to integrate into postmodern psychotherapy, several attempts have been made to do so. A prime example is the work of A. H. Almaas, who has initiated a therapeutic method based on translating traditional Sufi psychological maps, such as those dealing with *fana* and *nafs,* into Western language (Almaas, 1987, 1989, 1990). Another early theoretical foray bridging Sufism and Western psychology was the written work on this subject by Pir Vilayat Inayat Khan (1982), the son of Hazrat Inayat Khan.

Moving from theory to actual practice in the counseling environment, the late Murshid Moineddin Jablonski (the spiritual successor of Murshid Samuel Lewis) developed a method called "soulwork." For twenty years before his passing in 2001, Jablonski pursued a personal counseling practice using this method and also trained other facilitators in its use. In a series of sessions, the student or client is encouraged to establish a relationship with his or her own "spirit of guidance" or "high self" *(ruh).* This high self of the student/client, with the help of the facilitator/counselor, helps focus the session of dialogue with various aspects of the "basic selves" *(nafs).* The counselor/teacher helps maintain the clarity and spaciousness of the therapeutic atmosphere and intervenes to help the "meeting" of the various aspects of self occur in the most beneficial way. This new expression of the Sufi tradition in a counseling format shows one possibility for the integration of Sufi wisdom and psychology in the future.

The author's own work, which was described previously, has been named "lucid body and voice awareness." It represents a contribution of Sufism to the integrative field of somatic, or body-oriented, therapy and movement reeducation.

As mentioned at the beginning of this chapter, Sufis often hide their theory behind methods that seem simple or seem to intend to accomplish something other than transformation. Many Sufi practitioners also practice psychotherapy or somatic therapy without any overt disclosure that they are engaging in "Sufi psychology."

In this sense, one can see the elements of a Sufi approach to psychotherapy or somatic therapy in the following principles and strategies drawn from the practices above:

- Initial issues in transformation are centered on simple goals, such as recognizing diversity in feeling/somatic states.
- The student/client is encouraged to distinguish these states according to various methods, which harmonize with his or her strengths (initially) and weaknesses (secondarily).
- Experiments or interventions may include sensitivity to body awareness elements and centers, especially the heart center.
- Therapeutic goals aim toward the student/client discovering his or her purpose in life as a process of inner empowerment that focuses on the future as a motive force in life. This empowerment begins with a concentration on clearing a sense of somatic space within and creating a focused sense of clarity. Further developments again focus on the spiritual heart as a center of empowerment.
- Further goals aim toward the student/client experiencing healthy options for relating to self and others. These broaden the realm of possibilities for both the self and soul aspects of his or her being. One tests out one's realization first through "practice" with one's teacher/therapist—that is, within the therapeutic relationship. The work then broadens to the client's larger community and finally to the world at large, both human and natural.

- The heart awareness of the student/client is tested by its ability to be large enough to embrace more and more love for self and other. The heart usually goes through a stage of being "broken" as it confronts its own limitations and the limitations of its own self-concept. The heart then rediscovers itself, after various stages, as being part of the heart of Unity.

Through these elements and others, Sufism will continue to empower further developments in Western psychotherapy, whether these are recognized by the name "Sufi" or by the simple perception of their underlying basis, the translation of "Sufism": wisdom.

REFERENCES

Almaas, A.H. (1987, 1989, 1990). *Diamond Heart, I, II and III*. Berkeley: Diamond Books.

Barks, C. (1990). *Delicious Laughter: Rambunctious Teaching Stories from the Mathnawi of Jelaluddin Rumi*. Athens, GA: Maypop Books.

Barks, C. (1991). *Feeling the Shoulder of the Lion: Selected Poetry and Teaching Stories from the Mathnawi of Jelaluddin Rumi*. Putney, VT: Threshold Books.

Barks, C. (1993). *Birdsong*. Athens, GA: Maypop Books.

Cohn, A. (Producer and Director) (1972). *Dance to Glory: Samuel L. Lewis—An American Sufi Master* [Film]. Seattle, WA: PeaceWorks Publications, Peaceworks-INDUP, PO Box 55994, Seattle, WA 98155-0994, USA.

Cornell, Rkia E. (1999). *Early Sufi Women*. Louisville, KY: Fons Vitae.

Donaldson, R. (Ed.) (1991). *Sacred Unity: Further Steps to an Ecology of Mind*. New York: HarperCollins.

Douglas-Klotz, N. (1984). Sufi Approaches to Transformational Movement. *Somatics*, 5(1), p. 44.

Douglas-Klotz, N. (1995). *Desert Wisdom: Sacred Middle Eastern Writings from the Goddess Through the Sufis*. San Francisco: HarperSanFrancisco.

Elliot, J. K. (1996). *The Apocryphal Jesus: Legends of the Early Church*. Oxford: Oxford University Press.

Fox, Matthew (1983). *Meditations with Meister Eckhart*. Santa Fe: Bear & Company.

Friedlander, I. (1975). *The Whirling Dervishes*. New York: Collier Books.

The Holy Bible, King James Version (n.d.). London: Cambridge University Press.

Khan, Hazrat Inayat (1960). *The Sufi Message*, Volume 1: *The Way of Illumination*. Katwijk, Holland: Servire Publishers.

Khan, Hazrat Inayat (1962). *The Sufi Message*, Volume 5: *Spiritual Liberty*. Katwijk, Holland: Servire Publishers.

Khan, Pir Vilayat Inayat (1982). *Introducing Spirituality into Counseling and Therapy*. New Lebanon: Omega.

Lewis, S. L. (1986). *Sufi Vision and Initiation: Meetings with Remarkable Beings.* San Francisco: Sufi Islamia/Prophecy.

Lewis, S. L. (1991). *Spiritual Dance and Walk: An Introduction.* Seattle, WA: PeaceWorks.

Nasr, Seyyed Hossein (1968). *Man and Nature.* London: Allen and Unwin.

St. Denis, R. (1996). *Wisdom Comes Dancing: Selected Writings of Ruth St. Denis.* Seattle, WA: PeaceWorks.

Suhrawardi, Shahab-ud-din (1979). *The 'Awarif-u'l-Ma'arif.* H. Wilberforce Clarke, trans. (a prepublication of the 1891 edition). Lahore, Pakistan: Sh. Muhammad Ashraf.

Walker, Barbara (1983). *The Woman's Encyclopedia of Myths and Secrets.* San Francisco: HarperSanFrancisco.

TAOISM

The essence of Taoism has influenced Chinese thought and culture for over 2,500 years. Taoism teaches about living a simple life. *Ch'i* (vital life force), *wu wei* (effortless effort), and *yin-yang* (unity of opposites) are elements of psychospiritual healing found in the Taoist tradition. Taoist mind-body practices include diet and nutrition, acupuncture, and "meditation" or Ch'i Gung in its various forms. Taoist practices offer much for healing the mind-body relationship and psychospiritual healing. It is a path of nonattachment.

So many persons are psychologically disturbed by the many opposites confronting them on a daily basis. On a given day a certain person can be assured of money, love, and positive feelings. The next day one or all of those things can be lost. So we are tossed back and forth by our responses to life: one day we're elated; the next day we're in despair. Taoism teaches a path of peace that embraces the unity of opposites. Light and darkness, male and female, heaven and earth— each is an expression of the whole. The practitioner learns to find peace in their midst.

A popular Taoist story illustrates the alchemical elements within Taoist thought. The story tells us how the founder of Tai Ch'i Chu'an, Chang San-Feng, observed a fight between a bird and a snake. He learned that the hard and inflexible could be overcome by that which was soft and yielding. Lao Tzu wrote in the *Tao Te Ching:* "You see, what is yielding and weak overcomes what is hard and soft" (Kwok, Palmer, and Ramsey, 1993, p. 96).

Chinese medicine and acupuncture are being eagerly accepted in the Western world and, in fact, increasing numbers of persons prefer alternative healing practices to conventional medicine. It has much to offer the growing paradigm of integrative healing. We have much to learn from the healing practices of the East.

Dr. Tong brings a reputable background of experience in Taoist thought and practice. He has personally practiced and taught classical Yang Style Tai Ch'i Chu'an and Ch'i Gung healing practices for many years. His style of teaching offers the reader a direct experience of Taoist thought on psychological and spiritual healing.

Chapter 7

Taoist Mind-Body Resources for Psychological Health and Healing

Benjamin R. Tong

According to Chuang Tzu, that most venerable of Taoist sages, well-being for human beings involves something of a return to Nature. To be "natural" means observance of the following:

Do not seek fame. Do not make plans.
Do not be absorbed by activities.
Do not think that you know.
Be aware of all that is and dwell in the infinite.

Wander where there is no path.
Be all that heaven gave you, but act as though
you have received nothing. Be empty, that is all.

The mind of the cultivated person is like a mirror.
It grasps nothing. It expects nothing. It reflects
but does not hold. Therefore, the cultivated
person can act without effort.
(English and Feng, 1974: 156)*

You might well be wondering, Is any of this realistic in this day and age? Does one just throw schedules, calendars, and bills out the window? Are plans and goals not worthwhile? Do we simply jettison all concern for keeping up with the Information Age, shooting for pay

---

*I have taken the liberty of altering English and Feng's otherwise generally adequate translation of Chuang Tzu by substituting "cultivated person" for "perfect man." My choice, I would propose, is closer to the original text in Chinese.

raises, and investing in mutual funds? This style of wandering "where there is no path" and grasping at nothing sounds easy for Taoists subsisting on low overhead—sequestered away in high mountain anonymity, living off the land, and doing little more than deep breathing exercises.

I will present here a basic description of Taoism and the approach that this long-standing but inadequately understood tradition has taken with issues related to wellness, illness, and "treatment," for individuals as well as for entire societies.

TAOISM: THE TAO, CH'I, AND CH'I GUNG

The central concept in Taoism is Tao. (*Dao* is the romanticization of choice at this time in the People's Republic of China.) Although the long-standing everyday use of the word remains as "way," "road," or "path," the classical definition of Tao is the "universal life force"—the closest approximation to the Western notion of God. Essentially undefinable and ever changing, this all-pervasive force or energy is transcendent and immanent. Similar to Paul Tillich's metaphor for God, "the Ground of All Being," the Tao is in all that is, and stands over and against the whole of Creation.

The opening chapter of the Tao Te Ching, the central work of the 1,600-volume Taoist canon, informs us of the futility of any and all attempts to capture this force in finite cages of words:

> The Tao that can be told is not the eternal Tao.
> The name that can be named is not the eternal name.
> The nameless is the beginning of heaven and earth. . . .
> (Feng and English, 1972:1)

At the heart of the Tao is the quality of multiplicity: The force manifests itself in an infinite number of ways. Its two most fundamental expressions are the oppositional elements of yin and yang. In nature—which includes human nature—objects and organisms characterized by yin can be described as either weak, dark, moist, still, or cold, while a yang valence would mean such characteristics as strength, light, dryness, activity, or heat (Chang, 1975; Cleary, 1991; Tong, 1994).

Imagine a tree on a bright summer morning. That part of the tree touched by the sun's rays is called the yang side, while the side not affected by solar energy—the relatively cooler and darker aspect—is the tree's yin face. With the passage of time, the sun moves across the sky and what was previously the yang portion of the tree becomes the yin side, and vice versa. The ultimate in yangness is the sun: In Chinese, it is referred to as *tai yang,* the "Big Yang." The ultimate in yinness would be the utterly dark and cold regions of outer space.

Over the years, many have equated yin with the so-called "feminine principle" and yang with masculinity. According to my Taoist mentors, there is no such proposition in the Taoist canon. It cannot be emphasized enough that the ancient Taoists had no intention of establishing what can only be referred to as a blatantly sexist distinction. Men and women are *both* yin and yang, although in opposite ways.

For example, let us compare a man and a woman, holding constant as many bodily equivalents as possible. That is to say, both are the same relative to age, height, weight, ethnicity, and so forth. In most instances, the man's muscles, bones, and joints would be stronger than that of the woman. We may thus observe that his "yang force" is on the outside, while his "yin force" is on the inside. Conversely, a woman's "yang power" is on the inside: Only *she* has the awesome capacity within to sustain the life of another human being—an unborn child—and eventually, nine months down the line, send that new life out into the world. A man does not have such power.

Another view of the relationship between yin and yang is that of balance. To the extent that health and wellness involve dietary considerations, Taoist healers have cautioned against such conditions as "excess" and "deficiency" in yin and yang. When there is high consumption of fried, oily, or rich foods, the body is "over yang." In addition to skin problems, weight gain, and constipation, symptoms may also include irritability, difficulty with concentration, and sleep disorders. When the body is "over yin"—frequently the case with strict vegetarians as well as those who continually eat cold and raw foods—the person experiences frequent fatigue, intestinal cramps, susceptibility to assorted viruses, and general loss of motivation.

In addition to yin and yang, the Tao is also manifest in five quintessential processes represented by the emblems wood, fire, earth, metal, and water. The Theory of the Five Phases is a "system of correspondences and patterns that subsume events and things, especially in relationship to their dynamics" (Kaptchuk, 1983:343). Akin to the Buddhist idea that everything in the universe is intimately entwined with everything else, this paradigm represents the conceptual foundation of the Chinese health and healing arts. Modern people throw garbage in the sea and then wonder why the fish wash up poisoned and dead. Many push their minds and bodies to stressed extremes and are puzzled that they would develop all manner of life-threatening diseases and ailments. They have little sense of the profound interconnectedness of all that is.

The Five Phases Theory teaches us that both prevention and treatment in health practices require strict attention to the exact correspondences between organ systems and emotional states. For example, within the element of wood, difficulties with anger will impact on the liver system. Earth corresponds with the spleen, the energy of which is affected by chronic worry and excessive thinking. The vital energy of the lung system is like metal, and can be negatively influenced by prolonged sadness. Fear is known to deplete the waterlike energy of the kidneys. Most curious of all, the heart system, aligned with the element of fire, is strained by excesses of joy, desire, and passion.

Finally, in the human body itself, the Tao is present in the form of *Ch'i* (pronounced "chee") or vital energy. Each organ system as well as the blood has its own unique type of *Ch'i.* Moreover, *Ch'i* in its most refined form is found in *shen,* spiritual or wisdom energy, and *ch'ing,* sex energy. The former is located in the brain; the latter is in the kidneys. Everyone is born with a set amount of these refined varieties of *Ch'i,* some of us being more endowed than others.

Ch'i Gung (or qigong), in turn, refers to any and all disciplined activities that serve to strengthen, balance, or enhance *Ch'i,* the vital energy. There are four categories of Ch'i Gung (sometimes misleadingly called "meditative practices"): sitting, standing, lying down, and moving. In the West, Tai Ch'i Chu'an is the most well known of the moving Ch'i Gung forms (see Photo 7.1). The substantial medical health benefits of Ch'i Gung have been documented by clinical and experimental studies (Bian, 1987; Dong and Esser, 1990; Gao, 1997; Liang and Wu, 1997; Reid, 1996, 1998). Similarly, Ch'i Gung has been shown to be effective as well for treating select psychological problems, ranging from stress disorders to deep fears and anxiety (Bogart, 1991; Goleman, 1976a,b; Hammer, 1990).

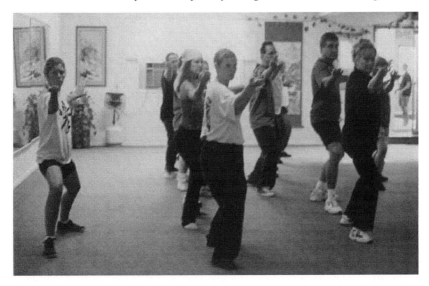

PHOTO 7.1. Tai Ch'i Class. Courtesy of Taoist Sanctuary in San Diego, California.

"GOOD-ENOUGH" HEALTH AND WELLNESS

Ordinarily, Taoists do not equate health and wellness with deep training under the tutelage of high masters atop steep mountains in monastic removal from everyday life. As recommended by my own Taoist mentors, a "good-enough" standard for most people consists of the following "bottom-line" principles: Sensible maintenance of mind and body, balanced emotions, an adequate amount of autonomy, and kindness to others. The key consideration in each instance is the cultivation of an attitude of nonattachment. Allow me to highlight an illustrative case study.

Many years ago, before the end of the Cold War, I was asked to provide stress management consultation to a group of high-ranking officers at a U.S. Air Force missile base. These military professionals had been experiencing a range of serious stress disorders. Given the excruciating pressure of career demands and day-to-day responsibilities on the job, their pressure-cooker situation was almost inevitable. I was reminded of similar conditions among air traffic controllers. As a colonel put it to me in an aside, "If we don't do something soon, more and more of us will drop like flies."

To make a long story short, I taught select Ch'i Gung exercises and, in addition, I made strategic use of an acronym from the technical vocabulary of the officers. At the time, all Air Force bases had what was known as the distant early warning, or DEW, system. This consisted of a series of systematic warning alarms on room-size high-tech maps to announce and track the approach of Soviet bombers toward target cities in the United States. This was the language of yellow, green, and red alerts.

Taking advantage of this shorthand device, I suggested that DEW should also stand for "Do less, eat less, want less." I emphasized the importance of attempting, each and every week, to find ways to actually do less on the job (e.g., "Is there something I am doing that really does not need to be done?" "Am I doing something that should be delegated to someone else?" "Am I doing something that another officer can actually do better?"). "Eat less" meant decreasing both quantity and quality of food ingested. They were to monitor the volume of their intake at each meal—with an eye toward eating "just enough and no more"—as well as lowering the amount of fat, oil, meat, and sodium content of dishes consumed. "Want less," finally, referred to learning to envision a viable existence if career dreams, worldly possessions, and the "perks" that usually go with high social status could not be attained. Through it all, then, the overall objective of "doing less, eating less, and wanting less" was to cultivate an attitude of nonattachment.

Lastly, I took a psychoneuroimmunological cue from the work of David McClelland, experimental psychologist at Harvard University, and encouraged the officers to find opportunities every week to perform or witness at least one genuinely kind and selfless act in the name of enhancing their own immune functioning. This was yet another variation on the theme of becoming increasingly nonattached—in this instance, becoming less preoccupied with one's own ego needs and concerns.

In one striking and still controversial study at Harvard, psychologist David McClelland showed students a film of Mother Teresa, the embodiment of altruism, working among Calcutta's sick and poor. Tests conducted after the film was viewed revealed an increase in Immunoglobulin A, an antibody that helps defend the body against respiratory infections. Even those students who said they didn't care for the saintly nun showed the enhanced immune response. Researchers aren't certain what the finding means, but it hints at a link between altruism and immunity (Growald-Rockefeller and Luks, 1988:53).

Bottom-line "good-enough" health, then, consists of centering one's day-to-day life around the theme of "less is more." An old Taoist teaching observes that "Our needs are few, but our wants are endless." When we simplify our existence—by developing ways to become less attached to possessions, desires, and activities—the returns for wellness are manifold.

The following story demonstrates the above Taoist healing principles with a woman suffering from a mysterious heart disease.

A very affluent San Francisco woman, Mary T., sought treatment with Dr. K.G. Chen, a Taoist practitioner of TCM (traditional Chinese medicine), a healer of reknown who at one time instructed her husband in the martial arts. Mary had been to a succession of cardiologists, complaining about chest pain, rapid and irregular heart rhythm, shortness of breath, etc., all the usual signs of cardiovascular disease.

Each of these Western specialists, however, informed her that she really didn't seem to have any medical problems with her heart. The symptoms were indeed something of a puzzle. Nonetheless, Mary was convinced that her days were truly numbered and could not see how these experts could be wrong: "Any day now I could have a heart attack, I swear!"

When Dr. Chen consented to meet with her, he asked that they meet at a Chinese vegetarian restaurant in the "New Chinatown" district of San Francisco. She was puzzled but decided it would be all right. Before the session, Dr. Chen phoned me and asked that I go along as an interested observer, especially since I was, at the time, in the middle of a research project on indigenous health and healers.

At our table, Dr. Chen proceeded to take a diagnostic assessment almost immediately. He read Mary's pulse and asked her detailed questions concerning her eating habits, lifestyle concerns, and relationships. Then he stopped and suggested that we order dinner and talk some more during the course of the meal. As we were wrapping up with mango pudding dessert, Mary looked Dr. Chen in the eye and asked, "Well, are those doctors right or wrong about my condition?"

Dr. Chen said, "They're wrong in their diagnosis that you do not have a heart problem, because you do."

Stunned and a bit beside herself, Mary struggled with a stuttered response: "Uh—what do you mean? What kind of problem do I have that escaped the eyes of those specialists?"

He paused and said nothing, which did not do much for Mary's composure. "Wait a second, please. Now, Dr. Tong here *also* has a heart condition."

"What!" I exclaimed, not expecting this unsolicited evaluation.

"I will get to you in a moment, but let me first address Mary's situation," he said with a disturbing calmness.

"Mary, first, I want you to pick up the check for this fine meal!" Puzzled, she said she would do just that. Dr. Chen went on: "Next, you can write me a personal check for five thousand dollars."

"What?" she screamed. "Now you really have me puzzled, even very suspicious! What in the world do you want that kind of money for? I was told you were a dedicated and nonmaterialistic healer of the first rank. So *what* are you doing?"

"The money isn't for me," Dr. Chen replied. "It is for people I will need to hire to climb the Chang Bai Shan [Ever White] Mountains in central China. They will gather rare herbs that are extremely difficult to obtain by ordinary means. It is exhausting and even highly risky work. You need those herbs as part of your treatment regimen."

She said, "Well, it isn't as though I don't have that kind of money, you understand. But how do I know who or what you *really* are? I mean, they told me you were extremely skilled and . . ."

"Enough!" he hollered. "Let me explain."

Mary stared angrily at the good doctor, the words barely getting out of her throat: "Explain what? You haven't told me a thing about what it is I have and why!"

Dr. Chen did indeed explain. "Mary, you do have a heart condition. It is one that Western doctors, however, cannot detect. Your heart energy, or ch'i, is cramped up and tighter than a boxer's fist. This is because you are an ungiving and stingy person, particularly with yourself as well as with your material resources. This condition will soon develop into an actual cardiovascular problem. I would say that without the treatment I propose to provide, your years ahead will not be many."

Distraught and totally perplexed, Mary said, "You said a moment ago that Dr. Tong here also has a heart problem. So why aren't you asking him to pick up the check? Why aren't you telling him to cut you a check for five thousand dollars?"

"Your problem can be resolved only if you are to let go of that emotional tightness and give more of yourself and your resources. And I do mean a whole lot more than you've been doing most of your life. As for Dr. Tong, *his* condition is the opposite of yours: He suffers from what Budddhist/Taoist healers call 'stupid kindness.' He gives too much of himself at times; he has trouble saying no to people who want his time and energy. Unlike you, he needs to hold back more and set limits on his generosity. No, the last thing I would ask of him is to grab the check for supper. Do you get my point?"

Apparently, Mary got the point. When last heard from, she was doing random acts of kindness. Her symptoms went away rather mysteriously in a matter of a few short months.

THE PATH OF NO-PATH:
SUCHNESS AND SIMPLICITY

Taoists emphasize that life is simply what it is. If there is indeed a grand design, our decidedly limited, finite minds lack the capacity to grasp it. All living beings are born; they live for a while, and then they die. Other than for a few basic givens, we really do not understand much else. In the interim between entry and exit in this earthly dimension, those human beings who would be serious about living naturally should endeavor to exist in much the same manner as plants and animals: simple, discrete, and without baggage. Health resides in not getting hung up on the necessary meaning or outcome of any event or behavior. Alan Watts (1994) reminds us of this path of suchness and simplicity in a marvelous story of old:

Once a upon a time there was a Chinese farmer whose horse ran away, and all the neighbors came around to commiserate that evening. "So sorry to hear your horse ran away. This is most unfortunate." The farmer said, "Maybe." The next day the horse came back bringing seven wild horses with it, and everybody came back in the evening and said, "Oh, isn't that lucky. What a great turn of events. You now have eight horses!" And he said,

"Maybe." The next day his son tried to break one of these horses and ride it but he was thrown and broke his leg, and they all said, "Oh dear, that's too bad." And he said, "Maybe." The following day the conscription offices came around to conscript people into the army, and they rejected his son because he had a broken leg. Again all the people came around and said, "Isn't that great!" And he said, "Maybe." (p. 157)

You and I live in a world that insists on holding fast to such distinctions as good and bad, fair and unfair, and success and failure. The Taoists insist, however, that nature in its suchness consists of a *unity of opposites*. Life is both good and bad, both fair and unfair, and so forth. Contrary to our widespread romanticism concerning wild animals, cute and cuddly tiger cubs are, at the same time, creatures who live by the savage law of tooth and claw. In the human realm, imprisoned killers on death row have risked their lives to build levies in flooded communities; saintly priests have molested choir boys; and genocidal dictators have been known to be loving parents.

Taoism calls into question the adequacy of all established consensual notions regarding health as well as disturbance or illness. Similar to its first cousin, Buddhism, this tradition emphasizes diminishing attachments and desire as the sine qua non of naturalness. In modern life, the essential character of the realized self is understood to be additive: You and I are presumably not acceptable, not even "real," lest we come to possess all the "right" things in life: e.g., intelligence, security, wealth, power, reputation, status symbols, goals, purpose, control, etc.

According to Philip Cushman, this contemporary self is the result of conditioning by a consumerist capitalist society that has produced for its insidious ends a painful emptiness in the individual. This is a chronically restless self "that seeks the experience of being continually filled up by consuming goods, calories, experiences, politicians, romantic partners, and empathic therapists in an attempt to combat the growing alienation and fragmentation of its era" (Cushman, 1990, p. 600).

Health from a Taoist perspective, however, involves adopting a nonacquisitive, minimalist, subtractive lifestyle—a sensibility perpetually struggling to let go of what is deemed desirable, including life itself. Huanchu Daoren, a Taoist writing in the late sixteenth century, observed that human life is made freer by minimization . . . if you party less, you avoid that much more frenzy, and if you speak less, you avoid that much more resentment. If you think less, your vital spirit doesn't get worn out, and if you are not clever, your wholeness can be preserved. Those who seek not to lessen daily but to increase daily are really fettering their lives. (1990, pp. 139-140)

Chuang Tzu reminds us that "the sparrow building its nest in the deep wood occupies but a single twig. The muskrat drinks only enough from the river to fill its belly" (Ma, 1988, p. 2). Lao Tzu, the alleged founder of Taoism, taught that attachment to acquisitiveness or winning is anything but healthy: "[I]t is best to be calm and free from greed and not celebrate victory. Those who celebrate victory are bloodthirsty, and the bloodthirsty cannot have their way in the world" (cited in Cleary, 1988, p. 5).

The cliché "Less is more," sums up this fundamental Taoist emphasis on the profound benefits of living in the simplest, least pretentious, most minimal fashion possible. Many years ago, my primary Taoist mentor addressed this concern by demonstrating, in graphic action, the most energy-efficient way of caring for the safety of one's automobile in a big city. "Most modern people," he said, "needlessly expend massive amounts of precious life force to keep others from stealing their cars. This is especially true of those who insist on owning the latest, the most stylish, the most expensive models. They install all kinds of sophisticated security alarm devices, pay intense attention to where they park, and wind up wearing out mind and body worrying about car thieves in the night. This kind of deep attachment represents what we in Chinese call *chun doh gik* [the height of stupidity]."

Without skipping a beat, he suddenly picked up a nearby sledgehammer and proceeded to pummel the body of my car. I screamed, "Hey, wait, what are you doing? You're wrecking my car!" Master Chan replied, "Nonsense. I am only defacing the hood and doors a bit. The engine and everything else inside works just fine." Bewildered and upset, I exclaimed, "What's your point?" The justification was rendered in remarkably calm tones: "The point should be obvious. You and I need cars only to get us from one place to another. And that is all. Everything else is extraneous and unnecessary. Now that your car *looks* like a wreck, no thief in his right mind would want to steal it. You can park it anywhere, anytime, without stressing yourself silly about what might happen to it."

"NO-IDENTITY IS TRUE IDENTITY"

The truest or core part of us, that which resonates to the Tao itself, is itself multiple in character. The healthy self is actually capable of being more than one self. The real self is anything but fixed. As such, the more genuinely free a person is, the more unpredictable he or she becomes. We can appreciate this long-standing notion by considering the origins of the Chinese zodiac.

When the Gregorian calendar rang in February 16, 1999, Chinese communities all over the world ushered in the year 4697 according to the Chinese lunar calendar. The latter is a system that arranges years in a twelve-year cycle, as most of us know, naming each of them after an animal. The year 1999 was the year of the hare or rabbit. The year 2000 was the year of the dragon, 2001 was the year of the snake, and 2002 is the year of the horse.

However, not too many people in our time know about the original or classical story concerning the significance of the twelve animals of the Chinese zodiac. Nowadays most of us are inclined to associate certain distinctive personality traits with specific birth years. Rabbits, for example, are said to be generally quick-witted and intelligent. Methodical, honest, and conscientious, they also make excellent communicators. Dragons are said to be endowed with energy, vitality, and strength. They are direct and difficult to control. Snakes are deep thinkers who trust more in their own sensitivity than in outside advice. The original narrative, by contrast, paints a very different—indeed contrary—picture.

It was told in days of old that when it came time for the Buddha to take leave of this earthly realm, he put out a call to all the animals to appear before Him. Only twelve bothered to show up. The turtle did not check in; neither did the giraffe, the walrus, the hawk, the frog, the alligator, the ostrich, or countless others.

"Well, I guess I have to make do with you twelve faithful ones," said the Buddha. "Human beings," He went on, "suffer more than they need to because they tend to get too fixed in their ways. Each of you will serve as a reminder to humankind that they must change whenever life requires them to stop being one way and start being another." There are times, then, to be as persistent as an ox. On other occasions, one might need to be as nimble as a monkey, or as fierce as a tiger, or as alert as a rooster, or as loyal as a dog, or as gentle as a sheep, or as independent as a boar, or as holy as a dragon, and so on.

This was more than just quaint folklore, for the central teaching was that attachment to an overly consistent or rigid sense of self causes us to "miss the mark"—to borrow from the original Greek archery definition of the concept of sin—in terms of appropriate ways of being with self, others, nature, and God. This resonates to the core metaphor of the famous Shaolin Temple in ancient China.

Shaolin means "eternally young wilderness." The highly evolved or cultivated person actually has many selves. Depending on the occasion, one can alternately become a horse, or a rat, or any of the twelve animals. One should not and need not be wedded to any one mode of response to the challenging and complex situations of life. The modern Taoist scholar, Chang Chung-Yuan, wrote that "no-identity is true identity" (1975, p. 26; see also Lifton, 1995; Gergen, 1994; Parry, 1991; Smith, 1994; Stroebe and Gergen, 1992). A clinical example illustrates further.

Susan M., a longtime professional colleague of mine, has the reputation of being a first-rate child psychotherapist in the San Francisco Bay Area. Her style is said to be Rogerian (after the master therapist Carl Rogers) or nondirective: She is usually subtle, attentive, soft-spoken, and indirect—exquisitely so. Some time ago, Susan struggled to help Candice, a fourteen-year-old adolescent client referred by a school counselor. Candice was in an unhealthy enmeshed relationship with her possessive mother, a socially isolated divorcée. A bright and high-achieving student, Candice had no life of her own apart from her academic studies and her mother. She was her mother's constant companion and confidante.

For weeks on end Susan tried every intervention consistent with her therapeutic approach and style, but things simply remained stuck at an impasse. One afternoon, Candice asked whether it would be all right for the two of them to leave Susan's office and go for a walk outside, in the midst of a light drizzle. Several minutes into their leisurely walk, Susan suddenly found herself doing something dramatic and completely without precedent. As she described the scenario to participants in a clinical training workshop, Susan said, "I found myself coming to a dead stop and spinning ninety degrees to face Candice squarely at close range. And then the words leaped out of my mouth: 'You have no business conducting your life like this. You need to let go of Mother and grow up and develop like a normal teenager. You really needn't worry about your mother, because she *will* be able to find her own way.'" Susan went on to disclose that she had never been so direct with a client: "It really was not me, and yet it was absolutely appropriate. Candice went on to do exactly as I had insisted."

My interpretation of this intriguing turn of events was that in asking for a change in therapeutic context (walking outside in the drizzle), Candice communicated to her therapist, perhaps unconsciously, that she wanted Susan to exercise a change in *her* usual presentation of self to the client (in this case, being more direct). From a Taoist perspective, both client and therapist were aware, each in her own way, that mired in stasis the self can be unbalanced and disturbingly stuck. Each needed to be a different self to return to the flow of life. Candice needed to be a more individuated self, which did not necessarily mean abandoning her mother altogether. Susan needed to be a more direct and authoritative therapist or mentor, at least at this moment. Both women, in fact, serve as a graphic illustration of the Buddha's reminder theme in the Chinese zodiac: Be the self that you need to be as required by the situation at hand, as opposed to remaining tenaciously committed to a self imposed by social obligation or neurotic circumstance.

From a Taoist point of view, health of the profoundest and hence rarest sort resides in affirmation of the "fullness of being" through such activity as timely revolt against the deadening fixity of "normal" social role obligations. In her impressive study titled *The Managed Heart: The Commercialization of Human Feelings* (1985), sociologist Arlie Hothschild found that female flight attendants developed serious psychiatric symptoms after many years of enforced smiling. She also discovered that male bill collectors whose jobs required them to appear continually angrier than they felt also suffered similar consequences. Play any part long enough and you run the very real danger of the mask becoming the face: You will not know one from the other after a while, and your outward expression becomes so fixed that the self within is also affected by the pathology.

Allow me to share a more personal illustration of the point. My primary Taoist mentor, Sifu (Chinese for "master") Kwong Kee Chan once raised a question to his students: "What really is the difference between a steak served to you on a heavy, expensive, fancy plate and the same piece of meat if it were thrown on the ground in back of a restaurant to become feast for dogs, alley cats, and hobos?"

My answer to the *sifu*'s essentially rhetorical question was: In one situation, an ordinary person would be keen on biting into the steak. In the other, he would very likely feel excruciating nausea at the thought of consuming the meat. Sifu Chan, of course, was not recommending dining with animals in back alleys. He was talking about the human tendency to assign hard and fast meanings to objects and events according to the socially defined frameworks surrounding our human reality and the profound consequences of such symbolic investments. These meanings, from a Taoist angle, are games—sometimes games we cannot escape playing. The critical issue is whether we take such games seriously.

Sifu Chan spoke on the heels of a specific experience: One spring day twenty years ago, I drove him eighty miles down Northern California's highway 280 from San Francisco to the University of California campus at Santa Cruz. He was scheduled to appear as a guest instructor in one of my classes. On this semidesolate highway, I found myself with a bloated bladder hankering to relieve itself. Whenever a road sign appeared on the far horizon, I would strain to read the words in a desperate search for a socially appropriate facility for urination.

Sifu suddenly turned to me and said, in a stern voice, "What are you doing?"

I replied, "Sifu, I'm trying to find a service station—a gas station. Anywhere. I'm dying to take a leak!"

"Stop the car right this instant and get out and piss on the roadside!" He bellowed. I was dumbfounded.

"What? Why should I do that?"

"The simplest, least, energy-demanding way to do anything *is* the best way. This is also known as the Taoist way."

Given my deep emotional attachment to well-established notions of how a college professor should conduct himself in public, he was not in the least bit surprised at my initial reaction to his perfectly reasonable suggestion. If anything, horrific visions flooded my head: I imagined students driving by, exclaiming, "Hey, Dr. Tong, what *are* you doing?"

I was too invested in the "proper" frame or context within which I felt urination should take place, instead of simply letting my bladder dictate more natural terms. The best way to eat, similarly, is simply to pick up food and eat. In physics, this would be called "the path of least action." In Taoism, it is called *wu wei*. I recall occasions in which well-intended people of high social standing practically gave themselves triple hernias because of their attachment to serving light desserts "correctly" in fancy, heavy dishes on exquisitely embroidered linen tablecloths, with elaborate sets of polished silverware, to the tune of "dinner music." When I mentioned this kind of scenario to Sifu, he said, "Hell, just give me a pair of chopsticks. Just think of the massive loss of life energy involved in making such an idiotic fuss."

I recall watching a Zen-oriented tennis instructor some years ago working with a group of rather self-conscious students. He called for one decidedly obese woman to present herself front and center for a demonstration. The woman was very reluctant, particularly since Public Broadcasting System (PBS) video cameras on the spot were recording the session for public consumption. Exercising considerable patience, he eventually persuaded her to volunteer. "I'd like for you to go to the opposite end of this court, and I will hit you a series of balls," he explained. "And I want you to simply hit each one back."

She was immediately flustered and insisted: "I—I can't hit anything at all! Why don't you use someone else?"

Puzzled, the instructor asked, "Why are you so certain you won't be able to return any of my volleys?"

She replied, "Can't you see what I am? Take a good look! It should be obvious!"

He said, "What should I be seeing when I look at you? You tell me."

With agonized embarrassment, she declared, "I'm a big fat rhinoceros! A rhino trying to play tennis!"

He then asked, "Who is your favorite tennis star?"

"Why, Billie Jean King, who else?" she replied. "I've followed every detail of her career, in fact."

The instructor suggested that she go to the opposite end of the court and for the next five minutes pretend she was her heroine, Billie Jean King.

"Oh, that's silly," she said. "I'm obviously anything but Billie Jean!"

"Never mind that," he gently replied. "I simply want you to play a light game of pretend, that's all. We won't keep score. For the next five minutes, you will not be the usual you, the 'fat rhino.' You will be Billie Jean King." When she overcame her initial resistance, the woman took her place on the court and, to everyone's amazement, hit back every ball directed at her.

Undue attachment to a fixed sense of self or identity keeps one from actualizing latent possibilities. In a similar vein, I ran a brief therapy group some years ago with seven extremely shy ("social phobic") heterosexual men for whom the word "no" was inundating.

That is, "no," in the context of being turned down for a social date by a woman, meant, in the men's eyes, that they were necessarily worthless and undesirable. They were "attached" to a fixed meaning for the word "no."

My strategy was to have each of them engage in what Taoist masters refer to as "defeat-ego" training, which is akin at least in principle to what the Zen-oriented tennis instructor employed. I was adamant that in between sessions everyone was to continually ask women out for dates, all the while tabulating the number of "yes" and "no" responses. When their anxiety levels shot up at the thought of this behavioral homework, I added such therapeutic adjuncts as sitting meditation and Ch'i Gung exercises involving visualization and deep breathing. In the early phase of treatment, the men simply bemoaned the number of negative replies they managed to collect.

In time, however, the meaning of the word began to shift. One man would announce, "Well, I got seven nos, but, hey, I came back to tell you all that I survived it. And not only that, I did get three yeses." Another man would say, with an equal amount of newfound pride, that he had even more "nos." Soon the number of "nos" came to represent, in the words of the men themselves, a "red badge of courage" and a "purple heart." Once it was clear that all of them could live with the word "no," that life would not end each time it was uttered by a woman, they were properly liberated to go on with their lives.

"No-identity is true identity." Those who cling tightly to what they feel life owes them run the risk of illness and disease. I remember conducting oral history research for a period of some fifteen years with colleagues and students in the Asian-American Studies Department at San Francisco State University. When we zeroed in on the earliest generation of Asian-American actors in Hollywood, one very gifted performer expressed to us that the so-called "big break" into mainstream American movies had continually eluded him. The record shows that he was very likely the first Asian American to have been nominated for the Academy Award for Best Supporting Actor. Still roundly frustrated but persistently hopeful in late middle age, he said, "I'm still waiting. Still doggedly waiting. I'm not giving in, dammit!"

A wise Taoist-like mentor of mine, Reverend Dr. James Chuck, once defined maturity as being satisfied and thankful for the cumulative experiences of life. "One should be able to look back in the later years of life, and say, 'I didn't get everything I wanted and life didn't turn out exactly the way I had hoped. But the way it did turn out was good enough. It had its moments. And I can live with that.'"

ILLNESS AS "STUCK" OR "ATTACHED" LIFE ENERGY

Nature is in perpetual motion and change. Health from a Taoist point of view is grounded in that most fundamental of principles. When the vital life energy, *Ch'i,* is moving smoothly and vigorously throughout the body and the bloodstream, the individual is in a state of high wellness. Health concerns arise whenever the ch'i is not moving. Psychological and lifestyle problems are frequently traceable to being stuck in repetitive thought, feeling, or behavior.

I recall one of my Tai Ch'i classmates of yesteryear, Jane R., stopping at a particular Tai Ch'i movement—known as Repulse Monkey—and staring at herself in the practice studio mirror. She was so deathly still that I approached her to ask if she was all right. She replied with both insight and alarm in her voice, "Look, in the mirror! *That's* how I'm leading my life!" Jane went on to explain that her Ch'i had not been flowing smoothly even though her Tai Ch'i movements "looked right." She was aware that she had been "running around the same circle repeatedly" in her attempts to resolve a relationship issue in her life.

The wife of one of my professional colleagues, a woman in her early forties, was recently reported for emotional and physical abuse of her only child. She was forcing her talented ten-year-old daughter to excel in advanced mathematics and to practice on the piano two or more hours a day. The woman's own mother had been equally ambitious and relentless about the "need" for *her* daughter to be of "Nobel prize quality." Across generations in many families, people are attached to repeating die-hard traditions with intense low-level mindlessness.

WU WEI: THE ULTIMATE ACHIEVEMENT IN TAOIST "WELLNESS"

One might well ask whether there is something beyond "good-enough" health and wellness Taoist practices. There is, indeed, a "gold standard," but, interestingly enough, it does not fit into any of our conventional definitions of wellness. This is related to a paradoxical theme in the Taoist understanding of the human condition. In the Tao Te Ching (Chapter 71), Lao Tzu observes that "If one is sick of sickness, then one is not sick. The sage is not sick because he is sick of sickness. Therefore he is not sick." The "sickness" Lao Tzu refers to is the human situation itself.

Taoism accepts as a given the fact that the human dimension is no big deal. As the title of one of Paul Watzlawick's books states it, *The Situation Is Hopeless, but Not Serious* (1993). If anything, terra firma is essentially an arena of perpetual suffering. (In the West, Søron Kierkegaard has used the term, "sickness unto death.") There is "hope," then, only until one becomes actually sick or weary of being human.

On the face of it, this might well appear to be a bohemian posture of stoic gloom and doom. Indeed, the noted contemporary Taoist writer and practitioner, Deng Ming-Dao has observed that being "implicitly anti-social," Taoism "has no place in any society. . . . It didn't really have a place in Chinese society. . . . [It] is for those people that have seen the limitations of social mores, the limitations of social ambition, and want to find an alternative" (quoted in Towler, 1996, p. 79).

Let me elaborate on the point by referring again to the notion of multiplicity, or fluidity of forms, as a quality of the natural. All that is of the Tao is ever changing. For thousands of years, high masters taught that there is but one fundamental, permanent, unchanging law in the universe: the Law of Impermanence. All that is is in continual flux, chaos, and change—sometimes perceptibly so; sometimes not. Stability is the exception, not the rule. Everything constructed by the human mind and human societies is essentially illusory in the sense that such "fictions" (e.g., identities, statuses, roles, histories, reputations, rituals, institutions, goals, purposes, meanings, etc.) may feel real but in fact they are like whispers in the wind. Those of us who would invest in, reify, or exalt any of these inevitably become candidates for disease.

Training in Taoist mind, body, and spirit disciplines has as its end point the cultivation or awakening of *wu wei,* that radically non-attached sensibility which enables one to be both in the world and yet detached from it." In an essay written in his twenties, Bruce Lee observed:

The phenomenon of wu-hsin, or "no-mindedness," is not a blank mind that shuts out all thoughts and emotions; nor is it simply calmness and quietness of mind . . . it is the "non-graspingness" of thoughts that mainly constitutes the principle of no mind. . . . No-mindedness is . . . being one in whom feeling is not sticky or blocked. It is a mind immune to emotional influences. . . . Thus wu wei is the art of the artless, the principle of no principle. (Cited in Little, 1997, pp. 123-124, 131)

If I were a Zen archer operating in the spirit of *wu wei,* I would arch my bow and aim the arrow at my target. I would shoot as best as I could, but only with "just enough" effort and no more. At the same time I would not be attached to the outcome—i.e., I would not be invested in hitting a bull's-eye. If it should happen, fine. If not, also fine. In either case, my feeling would be one of "no feeling." Herein lies the secret of true vitality. This is vividly portrayed in Karen Horney's description of the "wholeheartedness" of an extraordinary headwaiter, as cited in a book on Zen:

At dinner, at the table d'hote, I saw many faces, but few were expressive enough to fix my attention. However, the headwaiter interested me highly so that my eyes constantly followed him in all his movements. And indeed he was a remarkable being.

The guests who sat at the long table were about two hundred in number and it seems almost incredible when I say that nearly the whole of the attendance was performed by the headwaiter, since he put on and took off all the dishes while the other waiters only handed them to him and received them from him. During these proceedings nothing was spilled, no one was inconvenienced, but all went off lightly and nimbly as if by the operation of a spirit.

Thus, thousands of plates and dishes flew from his hands upon the table and, again, from his hands to the attendants behind him. Quite absorbed in his vocation, the whole man was nothing but eyes and hands and he merely opened his closed lips for short answers and directions. Then, he not only attended to the table, but to the orders for wine and the like, and so well remembered everything that when the meal was over, he knew everybody's score and took the money. (Horney, 1987, pp. 33-34)

Wu wei is contained in that cultivated attitude of nonattachment which in fact represents the resolution to the human predicament: Through training in Taoist disciplines, one aims at achieving a readiness to live fully in the moment *and,* at the same time, to let go of life in that very same instant. Put another way, in order to fully live—perhaps this can be viewed as "wellness" of an existentially profound sort—one must cultivate one's life to a fine-tuned point where one is prepared for an exit at any given moment.

We see historic examples not only in the Taoist masters but also in such figures as Gandhi, Martin Luther King Jr., the historical Jesus, and others. At the most "mature" points in their brief lives, they were fully in the moment, tilting the axis of history, *and* fully prepared for an encounter with nonbeing, with death. My Taoist mentor once said that the single most important line in *Hamlet* is: "The readiness is all" (Act V, scene ii). Therein lies the fullness of life, whether or not we choose to equate that with "wellness"—which, quite frankly, I am not inclined to do.

In the conventional wisdom, wellness is usually associated with being illness free, living long, having satisfying relationships, and enjoying a stable if not predictable lifestyle. By contrast, the Taoist theme of living naturally, particularly on a high spiritual level, involves all that is unpredictable, uncertain, mysterious, adventurous, and dangerous in life. This is obviously distinct from the "good-enough" standard of health and well-being.

ON TAOIST MASTERS AND STUDENTS

Those who would traverse the Taoist path as delineated by Chuang Tzu in the opening citation must begin with serious commitment to a *sifu* (pronounced "see foo"), i.e., a master, teacher, or mentor (Dao, 1990; Chanoff, 1987; Liu, 1997). Since the classical era in Chinese history, this relationship has been viewed as necessarily a lifelong proposition, not unlike that of a parent/offspring relationship. The student is forever loyal and grateful to the *sifu*. A teacher for one day is like a parent for a lifetime. Deep teachings course throughout one's body for the duration of a lifetime, much in the same manner that a mother's milk sustains the person for just as long a time. One is to be eternally grateful, therefore, and forever humble for such good karma.

A teacher, in turn, has the profound responsibility of sharing only that instruction for which the student is ready. This presupposes a special relationship in which a *sifu* gets to know a student extremely well in order that the timing of instruction might be both appropriate and effective. My primary Taoist mentor once observed: "Teach a student the wrong or inappropriate thing at the wrong time and you are in for disaster." Hence the traditional insistence on secrecy and thorough prescreening of candidates.

A *sifu,* a "completely and highly developed" human being, is a master of the sage arts, the health and healing arts, and the martial arts—sage, healer, and warrior. Although he or she can "treat" with acupuncture, herbs, Ch'i Gung, and other modalities, the emphasis of the work of a *sifu* is seldom on dealing with disorders, despite the fact that ordinary people have continually sought such help from Taoist masters.

CONCLUSION

The editor of this anthology said to me, in a personal communication, that we should let it be known that "spiritual traditions have treated psychological problems for thousands of years. We're helping to heal the split between these two paradigms. The development of psychological understanding also enhances spiritual work. They're siblings" (Mijares, personal communication, 1999). I do not entirely agree with this view. From an Asian perspective, this split was created by the West. It has never existed in Asian cultures, where the psychological and the spiritual are regarded to be one and the same. The resolution of, say, neurotic conflict, emotional deficiencies, or unresolved trauma *is* spiritual work. Spiritual work, moreover, is done both *away* from the world, in semimonastic high mountain seclusion, and *in* the world, in encounters with individuals and social forces.

Most moderns do not fully understand the thrust and the depth of Eastern traditions such as Taoism, Buddhism, and Zen. In addition to incomplete comprehension and outright distortion, contemporary people of both the East and West have appropriated these "paths" or "ways" in the service of improving such endeavors as tennis, sexuality, relationships, management skills, and salesmanship. More recently, medical and psychotherapeutic health practitioners have attempted to glean from these ancient wisdom techniques and procedures for lowering stress, alleviating pain, defeating disease, and delaying death. As I have indicated, Taoist practices do in fact lend themselves to such practical application.

The psychotherapist trained in Taoist disciplines can, whenever it is appropriate, incorporate into the treatment plan such regimens as Tai Ch'i Chu'an, Ch'i Gung, traditional Chinese medicine (TCM), spiritual interventions, and Taoist philosophy, in much the same manner that psychological assessment (testing) and medications would be useful as components of an integrated Western approach (Atwood and Martin, 1991; Bogart, 1991; Goleman, 1976a,b; Hammer, 1990; Recer, 1995) (see Photo 7.1).

At the same time, however, it should be understood that there is no such creature as "Taoist psychology" or "Taoist therapy." Taoist thought and practices may indeed enhance motorcycle riding, time management, organizational leadership, psychotherapy, and the like, but the heart of Taoism and Buddhism has little to do with such everyday worldly concerns. I have tried to distinguish between "good-enough" health and well-being—much of which can be sustained with the help of Taoist regimens, most especially Ch'i Gung, acupuncture, massage, and herbology—and high-level Taoist self-cultivation, which involves nothing less than whole lifestyle shifts and radical personal transformation.

REFERENCES

Atwood, J.D. and Martin, L. (1991). Putting Eastern Philosophies into Western Psychotherapies. *American Journal of Psychotherapy,* 45(3).

Bian Zhizhong (1987). *Daoist Health Preservation Exercises.* Beijing: China Reconstructs Press.

Bogart, G. (1991). The Use of Meditation in Psychotherapy: A Review of the Literature. *American Journal of Psychotherapy,* 45(3), 383-412.

Chang, Chung-Yuan (1975). *Tao: A New Way of Thinking.* New York: Harper and Row.

Chanoff, M. (1987). Transcending the Sword: Interview with Deng Ming-Dao. *East West: Journal of Healthy Living,* November-December: 66-67, 92.

Cleary, Thomas (Trans.) (1988). *The Art of War by Sun Tzu.* Boston: Shambhala.

Cleary, Thomas (Trans.) (1991). *The Essential Tao: An Initiation into the Heart of Taosim Through the Authentic Tao Te Ching and the Inner Teachings of*

Chuang-Tzu. San Francisco: HarperSan Francisco (a Division of HarperCollins, New York).

Cushman, P. (1990). Why the Self Is Empty: Toward a Historically Situated Psychology. *American Psychologist*, 45(5), 599-611.

Dao, Deng-Ming (1990). *The Scholar Warrior: An Introduction to the Tao in Everyday Life*. San Francisco: HarperSanFrancisco (a Division of HarperCollins).

Dong, P. and Esser, A.H. (1990). *Chi Gong: The Ancient Chinese Way to Health*. New York: Paragon House.

English, J. and Feng, Gia-Fu (1972). *Tao Te Ching*. New York: Vintage.

English, J. and Feng, Gia-Fu (1974). *Chuang Tzu: The Inner Chapters*. New York: Vintage.

Gao, Duo. (1997). *Chinese Medicine*. New York: Thunder's Mouth Press.

Gergen, K. (1994). Exploring the Postmodern. *American Psychologist*, 49(5), 412-416.

Goleman, D. (1976a). Meditation and Consciousness: An Asian Approach to Mental Health. *American Journal of Psychotherapy*, 30, 41-54.

Goleman, D. (1976b). Meditation Helps Break the Stress Spiral. *Psychology Today*, February.

Growald-Rockefeller, R.E. and Luks, A. (1988). Beyond Self: The Immunity of Samaritans. *American Health*, March, 51-53.

Hammer, L. (1990). *Dragon Rises, Red Bird Flies: Psychology and Chinese Medicine*. Barrytown, NY: Station Hill Press.

Horney, K. (1987). Free Associations and the Use of the Couch. In D. Ingram (Ed.), *Final Lectures* (pp. 33-34). New York: W.W. Norton.

Hothschild, A. (1985). *The Managed Heart: Commercialization of Human Feeling*. Berkeley: University of California.

Huanchu, Daoren (1990). *Back to Beginnings: Reflections on the Tao* (Trans. Thomas Cleary). Boston: Shambhala.

Kaptchuk, T.J. (1983). *The Web That Has No Weaver: Understanding Chinese Medicine*. New York: Congdon and Weed.

Kwok, M., Palmer, M., and Ramsey, J. (Trans.) (1993). *The Illustrated Tao Te Ching*. MA: Element Books.

Liang, Shou-Yu, and Wu, Wen-Ching (1997). *QiGong Empowerment: A Guide to Medical, Taoist, Buddhist, and Wushu Energy Cultivation*. East Providence, RI: Way of the Dragon Publishing.

Lifton, R. J. (1995). *The Protean Self: Human Resilience in an Age of Fragmentation*. New York: Basic Books.

Little, J. (Ed.) (1997). *Bruce Lee: The Tao of Gung Fu. A Study in the Way of Chinese Martial Art*. Boston: Charles E. Tuttle.

Liu, Hong (with Paul Perry) (1997). *Mastering Miracles: The Healing Art of Qi Gong As Taught by a Master*. New York: Time Warner Books.

Ma, M. (1988). Dear Reader. *Mountain of Heart and Mind*. Newsletter of the Institute for Cross-Cultural Research, San Francisco, 1(2).

Parry, A. (1991). A Universe of Stories. *Family Process,* 30, 37-54.

Recer, P. (1995). Tai Chi Keeps the Doctor Away, Research Says. *San Francisco Chronicle,* May 3, p. 11.

Reid, D.P. (1996). *The Shambhala Guide to Traditional Chinese Medicine.* Boston: Shambhala.

Reid, D.P. (1998). *Harnessing the Power of the Universe: A Complete Guide to the Principles and Practice of Chi-Gung.* Boston: Shambhala.

Smith, M.B. (1994). Selfhood at Risk: Postmodern Perils and the Perils of Postmodernism. *American Psychologist,* 49(5), 405-411.

Stroebe, M. and Gergen, K.J. (1992). Broken Hearts or Broken Bonds: Love and Death in Historical Perspective. *American Psychologist,* 47(10), 205-212.

Tong, B.R. (1994). Taoism: A Precursor of Chaos Theory. *Open Eye: A Publication of the California Institute of Integral Studies* (San Francisco), 11(1), 20-22.

Towler, S. (1996). *A Gathering of Cranes: Bringing the Tao to the West.* Eugene, OR: Abode of the Eternal Tao.

Watts, Alan (1994). Swimming Headless. In Mark Watts (Ed.), *Talking Zen: Written and Spoken by Alan Watts* (pp. 149-162). New York: Weatherhill.

Watzlawick, P. (1993). *The Situation Is Hopeless, but Not Serious (The Pursuit of Happiness).* New York: W.W. Norton.

YOGA AND HINDUISM

There is a Spirit, which is mind and life, light and truth and vast spaces. [It] contains all works and desires and all perfumes and all tastes. [It] enfolds the whole universe, and in silence is loving to all.

This is the Spirit that is in my heart, smaller than a grain of rice, or a grain or barley, or a grain of mustard-seed, or a grain of canary-seed, or the kernel of a grain of canary-seed.
This is the Spirit that is in my heart, greater than the earth, greater than the sky, greater than heaven itself, greater than all these worlds.

This is the Spirit that is in my heart, this is Brahman.

from the Chandogya Upanishad
(Radharishnan, 1953, p. 17)

For over 4,000 years, practitioners of Hinduism have studied and used the science of breath, physical postures, mantric sound, and other forms of spiritual practice to enhance human development and realize the Divine. This constitutes a substantial base of experiential and phenomenological research in the areas of mind-body healing and psychospiritual realization.

Hinduism contains the richest mythological lore of all the world's religions. The stories are intended to awaken the listener from his or her deep sleep of illusion *(maya)* and discover authentic nature. The creation stories tell of the Cosmic Dream. In the dream, Brahma awakens and the world manifests for a period of time. When Brahma disappears so does the universe. This state of nonmanifestation is called the "Night of Brahma." Brahma is both Creator and Divine Consciousness. This myth not only speaks of the creation of the universe but also alludes to the self discovering its Divine Nature. It affirms that *Tat Twam Asi* (thou art that) or *So Hum* (I am that).

Differences in temperament are also accounted for in these teachings. There are differing yogic practices designed for the various personality types; mental, emotional, or persons more physically inclined. For example, jnana yoga (inquiry and analysis) is for the intellectual. Hatha yoga (postures and breath) brings harmony to mind and body. Karma yoga (selfless service) is for those who relate more to physical action and work. Bhakti yoga (prayer, ceremony, and ritual) is for the devotional type of personality. Raja yoga is the study and control of the mind. Raja yoga includes physical control as well as mental control. It is the umbrella for restraints, observances, postures, *pranayama,* and all stages of meditation, including concentration, meditation, and *samadhi* (states of realization). All types eventually come to this developmental emphasis.

These topics will be addressed in Chapter 8 presented by Eleanor Criswell and Kartikeya Patel. Dr. Criswell has studied, practiced, taught, and authored books on Yoga for (somatic) mind-body healing and biofeedback. Dr. Patel is a native Indian and a respected teacher of Eastern philosophy and religion. Their chapter offers a unique blend of Eastern spirituality and its particular expression in Western culture.

Chapter 8

The Yoga Path:
Awakening from the Dream

Eleanor Criswell
Kartikeya C. Patel

According to the Brihadaranyaka Upanishad,

> Whoever worships another divinity than his self, thinking,
> "He is one, I am another," knows not. . . . One should worship
> with the thought that he is one's self, for therein all these be-
> come one. This self is the footprint of that All, for by it one
> knows the All—just as, verily, by following a footprint one may
> find cattle that have been lost. . . . One should reverence the self
> alone as dear. And he who reverences the self alone as dear—
> what he holds dear, verily, will not perish. (in Campbell, 1974,
> pp. 278-279)

How does one awaken from a dream to discover that he or she is divine? The Hindu traditions have developed a psychology of yoga that
reveals the way. As Swami Rama and colleagues (Rama, Ballentine,
and Hymes, 1979; Rama, Ballentine, and Ajaya, 1976) have noted,
yoga psychology and yogic practices are not recent inventions but
have been practiced, systematically explored, and perfected over
thousands of years by its masters and practitioners to help individuals
in attaining harmony and balance between the body and the mind to
achieve the highest potential.

INTRODUCTION

Many Westerners are familiar with yoga as a mind-body practice, but few understand its roots. Hinduism is not a monolithic tradition. First, the Arabs, and subsequently the Westerners, invented the blanket term *Hinduism* to cover many diverse traditions that have originated in the Indian subcontinent. Bhakti, yoga, Vedanta, and Tantra are just a few of these traditions that originated in the Indian subcontinent and were subsumed under Hinduism. This notwithstanding, however, these diverse traditions also share a running assumption—namely, that our psychological and physical discomforts spring from our sense of spiritual alienation and that these different traditions are but ways to address that alienation so that our fragmented being can be healed. Sri Ramakrishna, a nineteenth-century Hindu sage and practitioner of many religions, explained that just as a mother who has many children cooks different types of food to suit the psychophysical and spiritual makeup of different children, likewise, Hinduism presents one with many diverse paths of healing that heals one's fragmented being. Eastern traditions tell us that our day-to-day psychological issues and emotional distress need to be situated within a much larger context. Our greatest suffering manifests as a result of spiritual alienation. We are asleep, unaware of our true Self. The traditions suggest the various ways in which one can heal this sense of spiritual alienation.

In this chapter, the raja yoga tradition of Hinduism and how it helps us heal our fragmented being will be explored. Although yoga is a spiritual tradition within Hinduism, it is also considered a science, an educational process, and a contribution to psychospiritual development in psychotherapy.

Yoga is a Sanskrit word derived from the root *yuj. Yuj* means "to yoke" or "to unite." It signifies, in essence, the unification or reunification of the self with the Universal Self. (This unification seems necessary because we perceive ourselves to be separate from everything else.) It also denotes the reunification or integration of the person—mentally, physically, and emotionally. In its ultimate sense, yoga refers to the reunification of humankind with the universe or cosmic consciousness or the Absolute. It is the discipline and training of the embodied human being so that it evolves toward what it is capable of becoming. Yoga seeks to provide physical and mental training expe-

riences to further refine the soma (unified mind-body). Yogic practices are quite ancient; how ancient has been debated by many. By
some estimates yoga originated over 5,000 years ago. The practices
have been passed from teacher to student, from generation to generation—a process which continues to this day (Criswell, 1989).

There are many yogas—classic, contemporary, eclectic—there is a
yoga for everyone who practices it. Why? Whether Easterner, Westerner, or cross-cultural, no two people can duplicate the yogic orientation exactly. Some students work with a guru; some work alone. It
is important to find the way that most reflects each individual's inner
being (Criswell, 1989).

Among the approaches to yoga are hatha, raja, jnana, karma,
bhakti, and tantra. Hatha yoga is the way of self-transformation primarily through physical disciplines. Raja yoga is the approach that
uses chiefly mental disciplines, namely meditation. Jnana yoga emphasizes discriminative knowledge by which the real is distinguished
from the unreal or illusory (our numerous psychological projections
upon the canvas of the world). Karma yoga specializes in self-tran-
scending action in the world—in the form of selfless service. Bhakti
yoga is the way of love and devotion focusing on the higher reality
conceived as a divine personality. Tantra yoga is a nondualist approach that seeks to utilize all of human experience and convert it into
a trigger for self-transcendence. Thus, dissimilar to some more ascetic approaches, tantra yoga takes a positive view of the human body
and embodiment in general, and particularly acknowledges the hidden transformative potential of sexuality. All these approaches are attempts to leave the alienated state of existence marking conventional
life and to regain the sense of union with the ground of Being understood as Self-realization. Then, upon Self-realization, the person can
dedicate himself or herself to the welfare of all beings. This ideal is
most clearly expressed in Mahayana Buddhism in the form of the
bodhisattva doctrine. Bodhisattva is a Sanskrit term for "enlighten-
ment-being." In this case, the enlightened being is dedicated to the
welfare of all beings. This ideal is also expressed more recently in the
integral yoga of Sri Aurobindo.

The yogic tradition has recognized the importance of these specific yogic paths and consequently has offered specific explanations
of yoga related to a given path. For example, in his *Yoga-Sutras,*
Patanjali (in Prabhavananda and Isherwood, 1953) offers the raja

yoga explanation when he defines yoga as the prevention of the fluctuations of the mind-stuff (*yogah citta-vritti-nirodhah* I:2). Krishna offers another explanation when he defines yoga as skillful action (*yogah karmasu kausalam*). All are attempts to leave the alienated state of existence and regain the sense of union with the ground of Being. Further, the aim of these paths is to remove obstacles to self-expression and to help the self attain its freedom. Thus Patanjali maintains that yoga helps an individual to free the self of the restrictions imposed by the fluctuating consciousness and to attain the ultimate self-expression.

Chaudhuri (1975, p. 236) lists the following yoga disciplines which evolved from the fifth century B.C.E. to the eighteenth century C.E.: The yoga of breath control (hatha); the yoga of mind control (raja); the yoga of action (karma); the yoga of love (bhakti); the yoga of knowledge (jnana); the yoga of "being-energy" (kundalini); and the yoga of integral consciousness (purna). He says "the ultimate goal of all of the above self-disciplines is blissful union with the Self in its transcendental dimension of oneness with timeless Being." They are different in their approach, but they are all moving toward self-realization, freedom, and ego-transcendence. Chaudhuri's conception of "integral yoga" stresses the necessity of moving beyond development of the self to the use of that self in the development of society.

Integral yoga bridges the gap between transcendence and participation in the world. Chaudhuri describes *samadhi* as "the experience of freedom, immortality, transcendence of subject-object dichotomy, inexpressible bliss, limitless expansion of consciousness" (1975, p. 246). Immediately following self-realization, there is a brief period of inaction followed by a new kind of action. This action, empowered by being-energy, is used along the lines of one's perceived destiny. Chaudhuri (1975) says, "the unmistakable mark or this authentic self-realization [the individual's] would be his egoless dedication to cosmic welfare" (p. 252). The acceptance and interrelation of different forms of yoga has other implications as well. For example, this nonabsolutism also guarantees the differences in interpretation of what yoga, yogic *asanas* or postures, and yogic symbolism mean for different cultures. A Westerner's interpretation of yoga may be radically different than that of an Easterner. Indeed, Carl Jung (1996) had the following to say about the Eastern and Western differences of interpretation:

> You see, a Hindu is normal when he is not in this world. Therefore if you assimilate these symbols, if you get into Hindu mentality, you are just upside-down, you are all wrong. They have the unconscious above, we have it below. Everything is just the opposite. The south on all our maps is below, but in the East the south is above and the north below, and east and west are exchanged. It is quite the other way around. (p. 16)

What Jung is trying to point out is that the Eastern and Western minds are rooted in their specific traditions, and their interpretations consequently will be affected by these different traditions. This notwithstanding, however, Jung also points out that a Westerner, if sufficiently exposed to Eastern teachings, may unconsciously grasp the original meaning of symbols. As an example, Jung points to the experiences of one of his clients, a European woman who was born in India of European parents. In Jung's words,

> The patient was a girl born in India of European parents . . . the first six years of her life had been spent in India, where she had had a Malay nurse who was quite uneducated. There was no teaching of this sort, these things were completely unknown to her, but somehow these Eastern ideas got into her unconscious. . . . She could objectify the Indian psychology that had been grafted upon her with the milk she drank from that ayah and through the suggestions of her surroundings. (1996, p. 104)

Jung presented many different versions of this story in his different works, thus raising doubts about the authenticity of the story itself. Nevertheless, the important point that Jung made was that a person's unconscious can be affected by the host culture and consequently can affect a person's conscious choices, decisions, and behavior. Thus even though the cultural upbringing of different individuals may limit in the manner a person interprets yogic symbols, the unconscious makes it possible to understand and interpret the teachings with their original intent. More recently, increasing numbers of psychologists are demonstrating an active interest in yogic symbols, exercises, and their impact upon human consciousness.

Thousands of years of careful and systematic exploration have created the practical science of yoga; and although it ultimately formed into a metaphysical system, yoga is a prime historical example of an early science based on observation, projection of hypotheses, and experimental testing.

Most branches of Indian science did not experiment or test speculations (hypotheses). But Indian psychology—yoga—can be considered empirical in the original sense of the word: it is based on immediate experience. The Siva Samhita (Vasu, 1923), for example, maintains that it is only through the practice of teaching that success is obtained and it is only through practice that one attains liberation. The principles of yoga psychology were tested pragmatically. If individuals and small groups had similar experiences with certain recommended practices, if the effects were repeated generation after generation, if isolated practitioners reported similar results, then the knowledge could be said to have been validated empirically through experience.

As a science, yoga psychology most nearly paralleled science as it was known in the West from the time of Aristotle to the middle of the nineteenth century. This excludes the dubious contribution made by René Descartes to Western science: the separation of matter from spirit, mind from body. Yoga psychology entered the era of modern science in the 1920s with a unique event—the founding of the first laboratory devoted to the study of yoga at Kaivalyadhama in Lonavala, Poona, India (Funderburk, 1977).

Since that time there has been an increasing amount of Yoga research throughout the world: physiologists, medical researchers, and psychologists in various countries have been busily exploring the physical and mental effects of yoga using contemporary scientific methods. The development of technological advances and particularly the development in relatively recent (some thirty) years of the field of psychophysiology have enabled the physiological monitoring of yogic practices. Yoga and meditation are now considered a part of an applied field—clinical psychophysiology. From the unfolding of this field comes the use of biofeedback and self-control practices such as hypnosis, autogenic training, progressive relaxation, guided imagery, yoga, meditation, and others—all techniques that can alter psychophysiological functions (Barber, 1976).

The term "yoga psychology" is here used with particular reference to the model elaborated by Patanjali in his *Yoga-Sutra* (c. 200 C.E.). His model is known as "the yoga system" *(yoga-darshana)* and also goes by the name of raja yoga ("royal yoga"), the "eight-limbed yoga," or ashtanga yoga. Patanjali's systematization of the yogic path embodies the essential aspects of all types of yogas (Prabhavananda and Isherwood, 1953).

Raja yoga consists of eight limbs or eight categories of practices. The first two limbs concern an ethical and moral code: rules for behavior (behaviors to include and behaviors to avoid). The next three limbs are concerned with physical practices (hatha yoga)—postures, breathing patterns, and progressive relaxation. The final three are devoted to mind-training techniques: concentration, meditation, and *samadhi* or unification. These practices are thought to lead to the state of Self-realization, which Patanjali calls liberation *(kaivalya)*.

It is generally held that the body must first be trained before it can be possible to steady the mind, to make it focus. When the mind is able to remain focused on a selected meditation target long enough without distraction, the experience of *samadhi* becomes possible. *Samadhi* is the technique of achieving union with the object of meditation. At its deepest level this would be union with the Self. Patanjali calls this process "coincidence" *(samapatti)* between the meditating subject and the object of meditation.

In yoga psychology the mind-body problem has never existed (Chaudhuri, 1975). Mind and body are considered to have evolved or manifested out of the same primordial energy, *prakriti*. The physical environment is also thought to have evolved from the same transcendental energy source. Therefore, there is a continuity that includes all forms of subjective and objective existence. According to Patanjali, the Self or Spirit (called *purusha*) is radically different from *prakriti* and its various levels and forms. Whereas *prakriti* is inherently sentient, the *purusha* is pure consciousness.

Scholars debate whether this dualism is ontological or merely epistemological. The former is highly unsatisfactory, whereas the latter can be understood to be useful from a practical point of view. Most schools of yoga, at any rate, subscribe to one or the other type of nondualism. Thus the most common view is that although *prakriti* (material nature) and *purusha* (consciousness) need to be carefully held apart in the practice of the yogic disciplines, they are ultimately aspects of the same reality.

INDIAN SCIENCE

Science as we know and understand it was widely practiced in ancient India. Astronomy, mathematics, surgery, psychology, physiology, and logic were some of the areas in which the ancient Indians excelled. For instance, the Aryabhatiya, a book on astronomy, observed that the earth rotated on an axis. The Brahmasiddhanta discussed the lunar eclipse, solar eclipse, the calculation of the measures of poetry, instruments of observation, algebra, and so on. The scientific movement in India was not isolated from that of other parts of the world. Affected by it, affecting it, the scientific traditions of Western Asia and Greece related to it. In fact, as the eleventh-century Islamic scholar and historian Ahmad Alberuni observed, the scientific doctrines and findings in India had a close parlance to those of Greece (Sachau, 1971).

Indian science was compatible with a view of science based on rational principles. It entailed a rigorous examination of the claims put forth by many and acceptance of only those claims that passed the tests of validity. The Indians developed the theory of measurement *(pramana)* to validate a hypothesis. Briefly summarized, the theory of measurement asserts that a given hypothesis needs to be validated by specific examples; in order for it to be counted as valid knowledge, it needs to be proven. In other words, before a hypothesis becomes a conclusion, it needs to be argued for and validated by specific examples that prove that the hypothesis in question is an applicable proposition. The notion of measurement also presupposes independent validation of any data observed by the subject. It also presupposes the availability of independent and reliable means of investigation such as inference, reasoning, verbal testimony, perception, etc. Satischandra Vidyabhushana in his *A History of Indian Logic* (1988/1920), explains this theory of measurement with an example. Suppose a person makes a propositional assertion to the effect that there is a fire on the hill. To prove the validity of such an assertion, a person would engage in the following reasoning.

1. There is a fire on the hill (proposition or *pratijna*).
2. By our experience of working with and around fire in the kitchen, we can say that whatever has smoke has fire (example).

3. Because the hill has smoke (reason or *hetu*).
4. The hill has fire (conclusion).

A theory of measurement can suffer from many logical and psychological errors. It can be meaningless *(nirarthaka)*, unintelligible *(avijnatartha)*, evasive of the issue at hand *(viksepa)*, incoherent *(aparthaka)*, unnecessarily brief *(nyuna)*, unnecessarily broad *(adhika)*, and may contain other reasoning fallacies *(hetvabhasa)*. But dissimilar to the West, the Indian theory of knowledge was not limited to the knowledge gained through our usual sensory apparatus. The Indian theory of knowledge also dealt with other ways of knowing, such as extrasensory perception, direct, nonmediated knowledge, etc. The main tenet of the Indian theories of knowledge was that a hypothesis, however unusual it may be, can be admitted as a valid proposition if its worth can be proven with the use of specific examples. Our ordinary senses are not the only ways for us to know, understand, and communicate with the world. To summarize, Indian science sought natural explanations for observed phenomena. It had a theoretical logic against which to test ideas; and hypotheses would emerge from these observations.

Astronomy, physiology, medicine, and psychology were its most advanced branches of science; others less so. Indian psychology or yoga was the closest approximation to hypotheses testing. In yoga psychology (individual experiences allowing), body and mind training techniques are constantly used by numerous teachers and students to test yogic observations, principles, and traditional knowledge. Even today the yoga student is encouraged to test suggested practices in the light of his or her own experience. Cohesive, complete, intentionally all inclusive, early Hindu literature shows the results of Indian research toward an integrated metaphysical worldview.

Remaining in that state of static completion, hampered by constant invasions from outside and because of the waning patronage, Indian science did not develop further until the middle of its period of domination by Great Britain (late 1700s to 1950). Its renaissance period—an intellectual awakening—began during the nineteenth century. Indian science—through exchange of scholars, cooperative research projects, energetic exchange of literature—has increasingly identified with the contemporary worldwide scientific tradition.

YOGA AS SOMATIC SCIENCE

The methodology of yoga psychology can be divided into two categories: theoretical and experiential. The theoretical category includes the exploration of the essential nature of the human psyche. This exploration includes the careful observation, analysis, and evaluation of all aspects of human experience. The experiential category consists of various practices that are tremendously helpful in the gradual development of the self and self-realization (Chaudhuri, 1975). Yoga psychology is a highly accessible, organized system of mental and physical training procedures. It provides stimulation input for the following systems:

1. Central Nervous System: meditative practices
2. Sensory Systems:
   a. Vision: eye exercises, visual meditation targets, internal visual experiences
   b. Audition: chants, internal sounds, Indian music
   c. Olfaction: incense, perfumes and essential oils, flowers
   d. Taste: special candies, foods, and spices
   e. Touch: textures and massage
   f. Vestibular System: balancing and inverted postures
3. Respiratory System: breathing and breath-holding patterns
4. Cardiovascular System: various practices in combination
5. Somatic Nervous System (Sensorimotor System): active and static *asanas* (postures)
6. Gastrointestional System: fasting and special dietary recommendations
7. Autonomic Nervous System (Sympathetic and Parasympathetic Nervous System): all yoga practices
8. Ethics: the rules for personal and community-based conduct to realize the psychospiritual goals

In general, there is a movement toward homeostasis of the entire organism; there is, particularly, a shift toward greater ease in achieving parasympathetic nervous system activation and stress reduction. Yoga psychology claims to affect all aspects of the person: mental, physical, emotional, and spiritual. As a somatic science, all of these areas can be researched.

A particularly significant area of contemporary yoga research concerns the psychophysiological effects of yoga. Evidence of psychophysiological effects can be gathered from two sources: from research done specifically on yoga practices and from the research understandings of other fields (physiology, biochemistry, kinesiology, psychophysiology, psychology) which might shed light on the possible effects of yoga practices. This phenomenological analysis of yoga practices from a psychophysiological perspective could be the basis for further controlled studies to test hypotheses drawn from that analysis.

In a marvelous book called *Science Studies Yoga* (1977), James Funderburk has attempted to gather all contemporary yoga research without evaluating it. The studies mainly explore the third *(asana)*, fourth *(pranayama),* and seventh (meditation) limbs of raja yoga. The areas of research include the following:

- *Asana:* EMG (electromyographic or muscle activity) studies, measures of flexibility, pressure changes in internal cavities, and the effect of breath
- *Pranayama:* (respiratory responses): nostril dominance, respiratory pattern (breath rate, breath holding time, respiratory amplitude), air movement (tidal volume, minute ventilation, vital capacity), gaseous transfer. Circulatory response to hatha yoga: cardiovascular efficiency, blood-flow alterations, heart rate, heart control, blood pressure, blood composition. Endocrine and nervous system responses (secretory products, autonomic nervous system balance, EEG [electroencephalographic] changes).
- Meditation: muscular system responses during meditation, circulatory system responses during and after meditation, respiratory effects, and endocrine and nervous system responses to meditation (EEG during meditation).

YOGA EDUCATION

Ancient India adopted a system of psychospiritual training that spanned the whole life of the individual. The individual's life was divided into four stages with twenty-five years allocated to each stage. Most of the yogic training occurred during the *Brahmacharyashrama,* the first stage of the individual's life. The young mind and body is supple and can be effortlessly bent and stretched. The idea was to provide a solid foundation for the individual's growth to help him or her realize the ultimate potential. During this stage, a student would stay in a hermitage and be taught different yogas. This training combined theoretical knowledge of the scriptures with the experiential understanding of the main tenets of yoga. This knowledge and experience was then carried forward to the subsequent stages of life and perfected to its fullest extent.

Yogic development thus usually occurred in an educational, learning context rather than in a psychotherapeutic context. There was usually an accomplished teacher guiding the student or students. The events that occur in yogic development can be processed with the teacher. It does not have a pathological model. The growth and development of the student is the focus. It begins where the student is and progresses as the student progresses. There is a great benefit in approaching yogic development from this perspective. This means that we are working with the development of the student's potential rather than beginning with the deficiencies that may be perceived. Yoga has a positive thrust.

Patanjali's classical yoga is a valuable system for fostering human development. Classical yoga includes eight limbs or categories of practices. The eight limbs are

1. Observances *(niyamas);*
2. Rules of behavior *(yamas);*
3. Postures *(asanas);*
4. Control of breath *(pranayama);*
5. Withdrawal from the outside sensory world *(pratyahara);*
6. Concentration *(dharana);*
7. Meditation *(dhayana);* and
8. Nondual consciousness *(samadhi).*

Consider each of these eight limbs.

The practices begin by emphasizing the groundwork, which is the development of an ethical system: the *yamas* and *niyamas.* Rules for behavior, the *yamas* or abstentions, include noninjury, truthfulness, nontheft, spiritual conduct, and nongreed. Svatmarama, the author of the Hathayogapradipika, an eighteenth-century text, mentions (Sinh, 1980) the following rules of conduct *(yama):*

1. Nonviolence,
2. Truth,
3. Nonstealing,
4. Continence,
5. Forgiveness,
6. Endurance,
7. Compassion,
8. Meekness,
9. Sparing diet, and
10. Cleanliness.

The *niyamas* or observances include cleanliness, contentment, austerity, self-study, and attentiveness to God or the All of existence. Again, Svatmarama mentions the following observances *(niyama):*

1. Austerity,
2. Contentment,
3. Belief in the divine,
4. Charity,
5. Adoration of the divine,
6. Hearing discourses on the main tenets of yoga,
7. Shyness,
8. Intellect, and
9. Participation in the sacrificial *(yajna).*

Besides these rules of conduct and observances, the following conditions would help the yogi:

- Cleanliness
- Residence in a law-abiding and ethical locality
- Solitude

On the other hand, the following conditions hinder a yogi:

- Exertion
- Fanatic adherence to rules
- Anxiety
- Boastful public displays of spiritual practice
- Overeating
- Instability

The purport of these rules and observances is not to devise a controlled structure that curtails individual freedom but rather to offer guidance for spiritual growth. It is for this reason that Svatmarama maintains that fanatic adherence to rules could be detrimental to spiritual growth.

The postures or *asanas* are the third stage of yoga. From a psychological point of view, the *asanas* have another meaning in that this stage signifies that the aspirant has settled into his or her practice and that the wavering of mind (instability) has subsided. It typifies the yogi's determination, persistence, and courage. Further, the *asanas* are a link between the individual and the environment in that they are named after animals, trees, rivers, mountains, etc., to remind the individual of the environment. They also exhibit the specific qualities of nature that they are named after. Thus we find the tree pose, tortoise pose, elephant pose, sun salutation pose, peacock pose, lotus pose, etc. The *asanas* include the movements and postures of yoga.

The *pranayama* or control of breath refers to breathing exercises, but they are actually the redirection of the flow of *prana,* the primal energy. The *pranayamas* are of fundamental importance because the control of *prana* helps an individual to attain an undisturbed body and mind. According to hatha yogins, the fluctuations in consciousness result from the fluctuations of breath. Therefore, if the breath is controlled then the fluctuations in consciousness also will be controlled. The following passage from the *Yogavasistha Ramayana* (Bose, 1958) best explains this point:*

When the *prana* vibrates and is on the point of passing through the nerves, then there appears the mind full of its thought processes. But when the *prana* lies dormant in the hollow of the veins, then there is no manifestation of mind, and its processes and the cognitive functions do not operate. It is the vibration of the breath that manifests itself through the mind and causes the world appearance out of nothing. The cessation of the vibration of the breath means cessation of all cognitive functions. As a result of the vibration of breath, the cognitive function is set in motion similar to a top. (p. 20)

---

*This material has been translated and paraphrased from Sanskrit by Kartikeya Patel from Bose's original in Sanskrit.

As a top spins around when struck, so, roused by the vibration of breath, knowledge is manifested; and in order to stop the course of knowledge, it is necessary that the cause of knowledge should be first attacked. When the mind remains awake to the inner sense, while shut to all extraneous cognitive activities, we have the highest state. For the cessation of the mind the yogins control the breath through meditation in accordance with proper instructions. (p. 29)

Svatmarama corroborates the above observation: for whom the breathing has been controlled, the activities of the mind also have been controlled, and conversely, by whom the activities of the mind have been controlled, the breathing also has been controlled (Sinh, 1980).

Thus the control of breath has a very important place in yogic practice. *Pratyahara* is the practice of sense withdrawal or redirection of consciousness. Concentration is the fixing of attention; meditation is the nonverbal dialogue between meditator and focus of meditation; and *samadhi* is the attainment of nondual consciousness in which the subject-object, the self-other dichotomy, is deconstructed and unity is experienced.

THE GOALS OR OUTCOMES OF YOGA

The ultimate goal of yoga, excluding Patanjali's classical yoga, is union with the All. Ernest Wood, in his book *Yoga* (1962), feels that most aspirants to the yogic way are inclined to postpone the ultimate goal. Knowing that the light of it illumines the way, they content themselves with lesser goals. The lesser goals of the practice of yoga include: peace of mind and heart; power of will, love, and intellect; direct influence of mind upon the body and the world outside the body; psychic abilities of various kinds; control of mind and power of concentration; control of emotions (removal of worry, pride, anger, fear, lust, and greed); bodily health, suppleness, beauty, and longevity; and the prevention and removal of psychosomatic dangers and troubles (Wood, 1962).

Even though yoga training is usually done in an educational/developmental context, it can also be done in a therapeutic context. The majority of the therapeutic uses of yoga have to do with medical complaints such as hypertension, asthma, diabetes, and so forth. In India this may be done at an institute, such as the Yoga Institute, Santa Cruz (E), Bombay, or in clinical contexts. In the West this may be done in clinical contexts or by the growing number of yoga therapists working independently. Much of this is done in an educational setting, such as when a physician may refer the patient to take a yoga class to help with a particular stress-related complaint (see Photo 8.1).

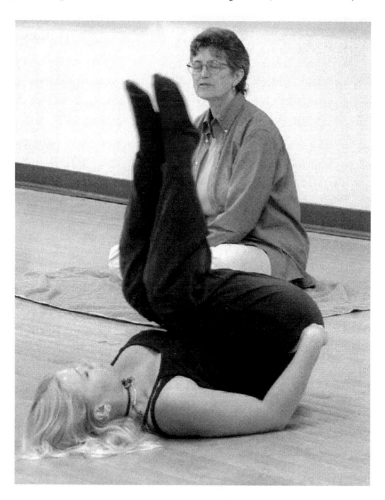

PHOTO 8.1. Student and Teacher Doing Yoga. Courtesy of B. J. Fundaro, Photographer, and Sonoma State University Media Services.

YOGA AND PSYCHOTHERAPY

Although not as likely in India, in the West there is a growing number of body-oriented psychotherapists who are including some form of somatic discipline as part of the therapeutic process. Yoga is one of the somatic disciplines often included today in the psychotherapeutic context.

According to James Kepner (1993), there are several structures for this inclusion: for example, the singular approach, in which the client goes to a yoga class or individual session and later in the week meets with the psychotherapist. The combination of psychotherapy and yoga enhance each other, but there is no attempt to interconnect the experiences. Another structure is the alternating approach, in which the client attends a yoga class or session and later a psychotherapy session. This allows for communication of insights gained during each experience. The third structure is the blended approach, in which the two processes occur during the same session. Yoga practice may spark psychotherapeutic insights, which may be discussed as they arise. A final approach must be achieved by the client in order to experience unification of the two approaches. The practitioner facilitates many of the client's insights, but many also take place within the client. Journal keeping of dreams and waking experiences is highly useful in this process.

Humanistic psychology has as its goal the actualization of positive human potential. This is usually considered to be mind, body, and spirit. It looks at the human being from the position of being centered within the human experience. It considers the spiritual dimension to be the further reaches of human potential and as a natural part of human experience. In the humanistic psychology context, yoga is seen as a tool for actualizing human potential. Transpersonal psychology, on the other hand, looks at the human being first from the transcendent perspective. Transpersonal psychology is psychology concerned with transcending the personal and frequently includes meditation, yoga, and other liberating disciplines as practices toward transcending the personal toward the human's true nature.

In mainstream psychotherapy, the goal of therapy may be personal adjustment, problem solving, resolving interpersonal issues, or the relief of psychological distress. Currently, mainstream psychotherapy is concerned with a diagnosis according to the *Diagnostic and*

Statistical Manual of Mental Disorders (DSM-IV) by the American Psychiatric Association (1994), and the formulation of a treatment plan that reflects clinical and experimental research findings. Humanistic psychotherapy and transpersonal psychotherapy begin with a different premise and move to include relevant experiences that unfold during work with the client. The humanistic or transpersonal psychotherapist would be more likely to appreciate the contribution of yoga to the psychotherapeutic process than would the traditional psychotherapist. However, other contemporary psychotherapists are also beginning to appreciate the contributions of yoga to their psychotherapeutic work.

The use of yoga in psychotherapy can happen in two ways: First the client can come for yoga-based psychotherapy with the clear intention of following that process. In this case he or she has usually been a student of yoga prior to beginning psychotherapy. Second, the desire to incorporate yoga may emerge as the client develops during the psychotherapeutic process. At some point in the therapy either the therapist may notice that what is emerging is relevant to yoga, or the client may mention the desire to take yoga classes.

Yoga in psychotherapy is very useful for stress management. Many psychological symptoms are intensified by intense and prolonged stress. Clients often have very few resources for stress management. Yoga makes a very effective package for stress management on a daily basis.

Many who are including the somatic dimension in psychotherapy are aware of the fact that merely talking about one's problems may not entirely resolve them. The client needs to be able to follow through on the insights, which he or she cannot do if the body's muscles are chronically contracted. Chronically contracted muscles restrict movement, contribute to pain, and discourage following through on intentions.

Yoga-based psychotherapy enables the person to develop somatically. The somatically free and comfortable body is receptive to psychospiritual experiences. In many cases the person is then able to understand and accept life situations when they are put in the larger perspective. A larger perspective is to be found in much of the literature on yoga, but it is more valuable to personally experience the results. The following case illustrates yoga in the psychotherapeutic context.

Marilyn was a sixty-three-year-old woman whose presenting problem was that she was distressed because things seemed to be moving around mysteriously. Things in her environment would disappear and then reappear. Objects would move as she watched them. She felt she might be psychokinetic. She had experienced a severe depression in 1975 which she overcame through a series of extensive letters to her brother who was undergoing Jungian analysis at the time. She was in a difficult marriage at the time, complicated by the alcohol dependence of her husband. She was also experiencing visual images of great intensity and beauty. She subsequently divorced her husband and moved with her two sons to San Francisco. She attended her first yoga class in 1976 at the invitation of a friend. Later she did yoga along with television yoga classes.

At the time of our initial meeting, she had a successful career in department stores sales. She had finished raising of her sons, lived well alone, and had mastered her trade. The moving objects seemed to be saying that "this is not all there is to life." She had the feeling that she wanted something to "happen," that she expected something to happen to her. She felt as though there was something within her that wanted to come out.

Weekly fifty-minute sessions were held over a period of several years. During those sessions, we worked with her dreams. We clarified the details; developed her associations to the dream material using personal, cultural, and archetypal associations where possible and appropriate; and placed our understanding of her dreams in the context of the issues that she was currently working with in her life. She continued her yoga practice; sometimes she attended my somatic yoga classes or workshops. She also began to paint some of her images in response to a heartfelt desire to do something creative. There had been a great deal of creativity in her family: her mother had been a New York vaudeville singer and a Christian Science healer. Her only brother was a brilliant publicist. She had been the appreciating sister in her brother's shadow. He was no longer living; it was time to develop her own potential.

During the course of her therapy, she was encouraged to take classes that might help her understand her experiences and life stage situations. Books were recommended or were found by her in her search for self-understanding. Her dreams were used as cues for areas to look at or new areas to develop. She tried to find personal meaning in her dreams and daily experiences. She read extensively in Jungian and related literature. She painted her inner visions beginning with a simple mandala that soon moved into more elaborate designs. The nature of her internal visual images is quite complex. Some of them are suggestive of mandala images of the Self; some seem to be synesthesia (auditory stimuli evoking visual images); some seem to be remote viewing; and some even seem to be precognitive, concerned with future events. When she paints from her inner visions, her paintings are highly sophisticated and quite beautiful. When she paints without the inspiration of her inner visions, her paintings are quite childlike and uninteresting. (Later she was described in a book on synesthesia by Richard Cytowic [1989], a neurologist, and interviewed on a national television program about Cytowic's research on synesthetes.)

She became very concerned with synchronicity in her life, trying to find the personal meaning in coincidences and letting them lead her toward additional insights. Daily yoga practice was an important part of her process.

My first goals for our work together were to come to understand her experience from her perspective and to help reduce her distress. The next goal was for her to learn as much about situations similar to hers as possible. (This she did through extensive reading, attending workshops and classes, and our in-session information exchanges where appropriate.) The third goal was to explore the meaning these experiences had for her. During the work on these goals, the degree of distress and neurological, medical, or psychiatric implications were monitored.

At this point in time, she has made a successful adjustment to this stage of her life. She has effectively retired from her department store position; she moved out of San Francisco to a nearby community; she has a part-time job as art director for a small special-interest magazine. She has recently begun a new enterprise: greeting cards featuring her paintings. She has a good handle on the tools necessary to facilitate her ongoing individuation process. She has learned to work well with her dreams through description, interpretation, and implementation.

She has also learned to manage her depression effectively, if and when it arises. She is working with her two sons very effectively as they go through their own developmental stage changes. Relating to her psychological process from psychospiritual, somatic, and psychotherapeutic perspectives made a significant contribution to her personal development and life adjustment.

Yoga and the psychospiritual dimension have increasing contributions to make to the psychotherapeutic process. It is a fascinating process, full of potential for expanded human function and health.

CAUTIONS FOR YOGA PRACTICE

Cautions for yoga practice concern the circumstances under which yoga would not be beneficial. For those persons who are psychotic or borderline, it may encourage hallucinatory experiences by lowering the physiological defenses they have developed.

Yoga can lead some individuals to dissociative experiences. It is valuable under certain circumstances to be able to dissociate, but it is equally valuable to be able to be alert and connected to the experience. Persons who have a tendency to withdraw may be encouraged in that direction by intense periods of meditation. Chaudhuri (1975) lists the following dangers on the path of yoga: (1) the danger of extreme introversion; (2) the danger of spiritual hedonism or gluttony; (3) the danger of regression; (4) the danger of emotional fixation on the guru; and (5) the danger of self-mutilation. In the case of yoga-based psychotherapy, the therapist can assess the degree to which the client would be a good candidate for a yoga-based psychotherapeutic approach.

YOGA AND THE PSYCHOSPIRITUAL CLIENT

Treatment Goals

Treatment goals for the psychospiritual client include the following: an increased understanding of the psychospiritual process; increased self-acceptance; increased ability to work and engage in leisure time activities and relationships; a decrease in fear and distress; an increase in the sense of one's life development and individuation; and an integration of the self-directed sense of this process. Increased understanding of the psychospiritual process includes the educational aspect of the therapeutic process. For example, the client may not know what a psychospiritual process is called or that it emerges in certain situations such as crises. It also includes recommended readings in the psychospiritual literature and attending workshops and classes from time to time. An increase in self-acceptance comes about as a result of the unconditional positive regard of the counselor and the model of acceptance of the client. Information about the nature of psychospiritual development is valuable for self-acceptance. Fear and distress often decrease as a result of the therapeutic process. The information about psychospiritual development gives it some grounding in reality; the calm, understanding attitude of the counselor serves to lower the arousal level of the client. This then reduces some of the fearsome elements of the experience.

The increase in sense of connection with one's life developmental course fostered by yoga gives the client a new sense of purpose in life experiences. It often gives an increase in a sense of joy in being connected with one's potential and life direction (one's Dharma), and reason for being. There may be a decrease in inhibition, which often accompanies acceptance and understanding along with an increase in available capacities and energy.

Treatment Plan

Yoga enhances psychological and physiological development, which enhances psychospiritual experience. Therefore the treatment plan for the psychospiritual client includes strategies for recognizing the psychospiritual experience. For example, during a psychospiritual experience, time, space, and causality may seem to be altered. Ways of enhancing and integrating the psychospiritual process may be appropriate, such as dreamwork, meditation, processing synchronicity and waking experiences, and education, along with other biotherapeutic procedures (for example, biofeedback). The therapist can validate the client's psychospiritual state during the therapeutic session and discuss ethics and contraindications. There is always a risk when enhancing psychospiritual functioning that ego inflation may result. Psychospiritual development needs to be fostered in an integrated fashion.

Principles from Jungian analysis are helpful in analyzing dreams and waking experiences suggestive of psychospiritual development. The principles include: clarification of the exact details of dreams or waking experiences; associations and amplifications at personal, cultural, and archetypical levels, if possible, developed regarding the elements of the dream or experience; and the meaning of the amplified dream or apparent psi experience placed in the context of the client's life situation.

Therapeutic Outcomes

Therapeutic outcomes include healthier, more comfortable functioning in the world. They also include increased self-understanding and self-esteem; the client should also be able to use his or her new skills in self-directed problem solving. Psychospiritual development needs to be comfortably integrated into life development and the process of individuation in life and sense of unification with existence.

Yoga practices and meditation have been considered psiconducive. *Psiconducive* refers to an experience that seems to foster psychic experiences. As persons perform the yoga practices they may notice an increase in synchronistic events. If they are not consistent in the yoga practice, the awareness of synchronistic experience may decrease or fluctuate. Often practitioners notice that they become more empathic with the emotions of others. Sensing what is going to happen, the yogic practitioner may even have an expanded knowledge of future events. The dreams may be seemingly more telepathic or precognitive. If as a byproduct of the yogic practice the client or student begins to experience what has been called paranormal experiences, he or she should be cautioned not to be afraid of these nonordinary states. Eventually, the expanded worldview can become the preferable state. For example, if the client dreams about the death of a loved one, this is cause for anguish. But if he or she sees life and death as part of the balance of the universe, then the foreknowledge of the transition of the loved one becomes cause for other actions and emotions.

If used properly, psi experiences can enhance development; if they are misused, they will get in the way of the yogic development. Misused, they will simply attach to the material world even more firmly—the world of material possessions and distress. As psychic abilities become more available, the *yamas* and *niyamas* as rules for balanced living in society become even more important. They can be helpful guides for the appropriate utilization of newfound or renewed capacities. Yoga has always cautioned against the misuse of paranormal abilities. Too often the practitioner becomes fixated in the phenomena, forgetting that paranormal abilities represent a stage below Self-realization.

YOGA AS A WAY OF LIFE

We have explored yoga psychology from both Western psychology's study of Eastern practices and from the research supporting the subjective experiences of vast numbers of people.

Yoga practice, no matter what the original goal was, will lead to the transformation of one's life context. Often yoga is a way of life for both the therapist and the client. It is beneficial for all to practice, for it unites mind and body while offering integrative healing and balance in the lives of its practitioners.

As we begin to take our development and psychophysiological maintenance into our own hands, there is the thrill of being master of our fate, captain of the ship. There is a great expansion of the sense that we can do practically anything we want to do because we feel an increase of personal power, well-being, and peace.

Our society has been experiencing rapid technological evolution. We cannot continue to evolve at this rate. Our planet does not have limitless resources; our population cannot continue to expand at its accelerating pace. The struggle to "make it" in our society has to become less crucial; we have to find ways to relax into our world. Educators and psychotherapists need to enhance the lives of those they serve. One way of doing this is through yoga and other psycho-spiritual practices. Yoga can help us relax and enjoy our lives, to really see, hear, taste, and savor our experiences rather than substitute quantity of experience for quality.

In modern times, we have become alienated from our environment. We have even become self-conscious about our alienation. Perhaps it will be possible to do something about it. We can hope so. There is still time. Yoga is an excellent way to begin to get back in touch with nature. It is, in fact, a way of establishing a harmonious rhythm with the forces of nature. As we begin to be more conscious of the air we breathe, for example, we automatically seek more pranic air. When we begin to do our yoga outdoors, we begin to feel the Earth and its more organismic sensations. As our senses become more refined and we begin to clearly see and sense our relationship to the environment, we will begin to appreciate more of what the natural world has to offer.

Some people who study yoga experience its benefits, but drift away from it over time. Others gradually incorporate it into their ways of life. Some individuals find it meaningful to devote their lives to yoga.

In India, there are various stages of life during which the person is devoted the dharma of that stage. During one's householder stage, one marries, has a family, and participates in the business affairs of the town or village. Later the individual may leave the ordinary life to seek philosophic and spiritual seclusion. Women and men follow similar paths with different responsibilities. Some individuals who feel their lives growing simpler as they come closer to the yogic way may choose a life of abstention. Ideally, this is done because the results of yoga become so splendid that it is not a sacrifice, but an advancement toward what seems to be far more fulfilling. We can make an intellectual decision to live a more ascetic life or we can follow the natural trends inherent in our development.

Whether we are in the East or West, if we are in the householder period of our lives, we are deeply involved with our family, friends, and society. This worldly period must be experienced fully in order to learn from it. During this period, yoga can be an integral part of our lives, facilitating our daily activities and fostering psychospiritual development. At this stage one is a karma yogi or yogini, living a life of service. May we all be happy and healthy as we do our work in the world!

REFERENCES

American Psychiatric Association (1994). *Diagnostic and Statistical Manual of Mental Disorders,* Fourth Edition. Washington, DC: Author.

Barber, T.S. (1975/1976). Introduction. Temperature Biofeedback, Hypnosis, Yoga and Relaxation. In Barber, T.X., DiCara, L.V., Kamiya, J., Miller, N.E., Shapiro, D., and Stoyva, J. (Eds.), *Biofeedback and Self-Control* (pp. xiii-xxix). Chicago: Aldine Publishing Company.

Bose, D.N. (1958). *Yogavasistha Ramayana* (Trans.), 2 Volumes. Calcutta: Oriental Publishing Company.

Campbell, J. (1974). *The Mythic Image.* Princeton, NJ: Princeton University Press.

Chaudhuri, H. (1975). Yoga Psychology. In Tart, C. (Ed.), *Transpersonal Psychologies* (pp. 231-280). New York: Harper and Row.

Criswell, E. (1989). *How Yoga Works: An Introduction to Somatic Yoga.* Novato, CA: Freeperson Press.

Cytowic, R. (1989). *Synesthesia: A Union of the Senses.* New York: Springer-Verlag.

Funderburk, J. (1977). *Science Studies Yoga: A Review of Physiological Data.* Honesdale, PA: Himalayan International Institute of Yoga Science and Philosophy.

Jung, Carl (1996). In Sonu Shamdasani (Ed.), *The Psychology of Kundalini Yoga.* Princeton, NJ: Princeton University Press.

Kepner, J.I. (1993). *Body Process: Working with the Body in Psychotherapy.* San Francisco: Jossey-Bass.

Prabhavananda, Swami and Isherwood, C. (1953). *How to Know God: The Yoga Aphorisms of Patanjali.* New York: Signet Books.

Radharishnan, S. (1953). *The Principal Upanishads* (Trans.). London: Allen Unwin.

Rama, Swami, Ballentine, R., and Ajaya, Swami (1976). *Yoga and Psychotherapy.* Honesdale, PA: Himalayan Institute Press.

Rama, Swami, Ballentine, R., and Hymes, A. (1979). *Science of Breath.* Honesdale, PA: Himalayan Institute Press.

Sachau, E. (1971). *Alberuni's India* (Trans.). New York: W.W. Norton.

Sinh, P. (1980) (Trans.). *The Hatha Yoga Pradipika.* New Delhi: Oriental Books. First version 1915.

Vasu, S.C. (1923). *Siva Samhita.* Allahabad: Panini.

Vidyabhushana, Satischandra (1988). *A History of Indian Logic.* New Delhi: Motilal Banarasidass. First version 1920.

Wood, E. (1962). *Yoga.* Harmsdworth, Middlesex, England: Penguin Books. First version 1959.

Conclusion

Each author in this book has offered his or her unique perspective and has contributed to a chorus of ancient wisdom on the topic of psychospiritual healing. The preceding chapters supported the premise that the search for our souls is the supreme undertaking. Integrative healing is incomplete without in-depth application of spiritual wisdom.

For thousands of years, poets, philosophers, and mystics have spoken of the longing of the heart to know reunification with the Beloved, unity with the Divine. After the long history of separation between scientific and religious thought, influenced by Cartesian dualism (Varela, Thompson, and Rosch, 1993), universities across the nation have begun to include spirituality in psychiatric and psychological training programs. The time is ripe for psychology and religion to blend the best of each tradition. As a result, psychotherapists and spiritual guides will be more effective in their work with clients. This integration will have a positive effect upon physical, emotional, mental, and spiritual well-being: the core principles of integrative health.

Spiritual teachers have been trained in ways to heal the soul. Psychotherapists have been primarily trained to diagnose and treat symptoms while ignoring the deeper needs of the individuals they work with. Therefore, it's time to go beyond applying temporary bandages to control the symptoms that loudly proclaim "Something is wrong . . . or missing." The symptoms often reappear once the bandage is removed. Psychopharmacological medications will not heal our minds or bodies. Something more is needed. This anthology states that this mysterious "something" is the spiritual essence manifesting in the inner core of life. It also illustrates the many paths to God, supporting a paradigm that honors all spiritual paths. In their book *Beyond Diversities: Reflections on Revelations,* Ali Rafea, Aliaa Rafea, and Aisha Rafea (2000) discuss the world's religious traditions and note that

> all revelations relate between how man approaches his earthly activities and his inner gains to realize spiritually fruitful life. He

should train himself to make all his feelings and actions stem-
ming from his higher Self and not the lower self. The shared
moral codes of not lying, stealing, killing, cheating, envying . . .
etc., empower the higher Self. All revelations call for love, cooperation, forgiveness, honoring father and mother . . . etc., to support man in his way to develop spiritually. (pp. 123-124)

The psychological contributions of psychoanalytic, behavioral,
cognitive, humanistic, and narrative therapies during the past 100
years provide methods for understanding and healing human behavior. These methods (Fadiman and Frager, 1994; Engler, 1999) can
help us actualize core spiritual values as psychological healing enables a healthier relationship with life. The developmental and cultural influences of our childhood are deeply entrenched. The various
psychotherapies are designed to help us go beyond the defense mechanisms that squelch our inner and outer lives. Psychotherapists and
spiritual teachers can work together to promote individual and community healing.

We can no longer isolate ourselves into separate groups, each pre-
tending to have the ultimate answer. Both psychology and religion
are undergoing major change. For example, the eclectic view of psychotherapy is becoming more acceptable. Clients differ in nature and
difficulties, therefore a therapist needs to be more flexible. Also, in
this age of rapid communication systems and the Internet, we are becoming increasingly aware and accepting of religious, ethnic, and
cultural differences. A couple of decades ago an interfaith gathering
meant that Baptists, Methodists, and similar Christian traditions were
starting to dialogue with one another. More recently, interfaith dialogues include members of the Jewish, Buddhist, Christian, Islamic,
Native American, and other wisdom traditions. These dialogues encourage us to live in harmony with our neighbors. They also represent
a beginning movement toward appreciating the differences and distinctions found in all religions and the persons following their teachings (Khan, 1979).

As demonstrated by the examples in this anthology, psychotherapy
and spiritual practice can coexist. The combination offers a larger
paradigm to the many individuals seeking psychological healing and
hoping to find a therapist with a spiritual orientation.

Spiritual beliefs and practices offer persons far more hopefulness about their lives than the biomedical paradigm suggested by managed care practices. For example, a male enters the office presenting a history of despair and failed relationships.

The therapist can give him an Axis I diagnosis of depression or an anxiety disorder and perhaps find cause for an Axis II personality disorder (dependent upon types of symptoms and length of time). The next step would be to refer him to a psychiatrist for antidepressants and develop a program to reduce the symptoms.

Or the therapist can present a very different view of the client's experience, one that offers a reconnection with the source of life. When the problem is viewed as one of a loss of connection to one's core identity and greater meaning in life, spiritual practices can help the individual awaken those forces.

Once we experience spiritual realization, we are never the same again. Life problems are forever after viewed in a different context, and we no longer identify ourselves in limiting terms. We know experientially that we are more than the problems that have plagued our lives, and daily life takes on greater meaning.

WAYS OF PRESENTING SPIRITUAL TEACHINGS

How does a person who hasn't received training in a specific spiritual tradition ethically present and apply the examples given in this anthology?

Each one of us has to find a paradigm that fits with our personalities, experiences, and related beliefs. Authors in this anthology introduced readers to a variety of experiential ways of working with clients. (Practitioners desiring more knowledge are advised to seek further training in specific traditions.) Spiritual practices begin to awaken the practitioner's finer sensibilities, and true realization begins. When people are authentically in touch with their deepest and truest nature and experience spiritual realization, their lives are forever changed.

Regardless of the model we follow, it is important to hold a deep belief in our ability to work through the tasks that life has given us. The belief that our clients and students are "more than their problems" offers them something that they may not have experienced before: many persons are suffering because of a lack of connection with themselves, others, and life. They need therapists and guides that believe in them; people who are able to see and mirror back an image of the soul. Many persons easily relate to life as a psychospiritual journey. Each experience adds to our development, leading us toward greater spiritual realization. Problems become blessings in disguise rather than symptoms to be nullified with drugs. A "problem" can open the door to a deeper connection with life and its wisdom paths.

There are a variety of ways to present spiritual teachings in psychotherapy. In the beginning of this book I mentioned life as a heroic journey. The following is an example of how I use this focus in my private practice. I work primarily with clients who have experienced some form of abuse or neglect in early life. When applicable, I tell a client about Carl Jung's theory on amnesic repression. Jung (1964) felt this repression blocked the natural spontaneity and creative power available to all life. Jung's theory was that life is a path of individuation, leading to the emergence of the Self. When clients release the block, they also release these life potentials, and life takes on greater meaning. Given this image, clients can consider the idea that there is something greater than the pain, anger, or depression that have them fixated in the past.

With this greater image in mind, we can move on to a discussion of Joseph Campbell's (1949) research regarding the world's mythologies, specifically those related to life as a heroic journey with four specific stages. These stages do not necessarily appear in a hierarchical form. I prefer to present them as spiraling paths, dipping in and out of various experiential stages. (I may not find it necessary to verbally express these archetypal stages of growth to my clients, but I am aware of their significance in the healing process.)

The first stage is The Call in which one awakens to the journey. Distress itself alerts us that something is amiss. I sometimes discuss the similarity in the stories of the births of Jesus and Krishna. Both had to be taken from the place of their birth to protect them from danger (Jesus was taken into Egypt to avoid Herod's death threat; Krishna's parents hid him with cow herders to protect his life).

I find it useful to use these spiritual examples as metaphors for the loss of authentic Self and one's center when abuse occurs (Mijares, 1995, 1997). Also, often a child makes a decision about himself or herself with inadequate cognitive development. Faulty core schemas can develop in response to one remark from a parent, teacher, or peer, resulting in lifelong patterns of poor relationship to self and others. A coping personality style develops, and defense mechanisms create further disconnection from authentic Self and significant others.

This psychospiritual theory assures clients that they are much more than their symptoms of distress. They are engaged in an archetypal, universal drama. The archetypal paradigm gives the healing process a much deeper intention.

Next I might tell clients about The Challenge, the second step, beckoning them to embark upon the journey of healing that leads to authenticity (a natural birthright). If it is compatible with their spiritual orientation, I often share Tibetan beliefs related to the afterlife *(Bhardo)* experience. In Tibetan Buddhism it is believed that the individual is tempted, taunted, etc., by false images that keep the person from recognizing his or her true nature. Isn't this also a metaphor for what happens to persons haunted by self-doubt, self-defeating voices, and other ghosts of the past? The Tibetan practitioner is guided not to fall into the traps of these illusions and experience liberation through recognizing true nature. The goal is to hold to one's sense of spiritual identity and to know liberation from symptoms and introjected identities related to abuse. This metaphor offers challenge and meaningfulness to what was previously viewed as a plague.

The third stage is The Initiation leading to the attainment of body wisdom. I often teach spiritually focused practices using breath, mantra, prayer, and meditation. This is practiced in the office and then given as homework. These are practices similar to those presented by authors in this anthology. My training is in Sufi practices and women's spirituality, so I often share practices and stories from these traditions. The person begins to improve quickly as the body and mind reach a greater sense of harmony. The client's identity begins to change. They are no longer bound by limited stories of themselves.

The results take one to the fourth stage, The Return. This is the place in which the client returns to a more authentic sense of self. This is the reconnection with life and the community. The person wants to share what they have learned and in some way benefit others. This process is also compatible with Alfred Adler's theory (Engler, 1999) that true psychological health manifests in our contributions to the society in which we live. Clients and students may find that career changes, family healing, and/or creative openings are occurring in their lives—affirming that transformation has occurred.

ETHICAL CONCERNS

What are the guidelines to follow when using spiritual practices for psychological healing? How do we implement the ancient wisdom shared throughout the chapters of this anthology? The various chapters offered brief introductions illustrating how each tradition treats psychospiritual healing.

Many readers may lack familiarity with experiential spiritual practice. The same ethical guidelines given to professional psychotherapists are applicable. For example, one shouldn't teach a method without adequate training and supervision. Professional psychotherapists are expected to recognize and honor the needs of the client. We are ethically aware of the scope of our practice. If therapists lack training in a certain treatment area, it is recommended that they either refer clients to another therapist who specializes in a specific field or that they seek further training.

In the realm of spiritual teachings, it is important to have a solid foundation. Authenticity is a necessity. This means that the therapist or teacher should have received in-depth training from a recognized teacher. The authors of this anthology have dedicated their lives to practicing the ancient wisdoms represented in each chapter. The depth of the knowledge and experience did not suddenly appear as a result of one or more weekend workshops or through the reading of a few books in a particular area. Rather this wisdom was learned under the guidance and teachings of wise teachers, along with years of study and experiential practice. Both the Native American and Taoist authors specifically noted the danger and disrespect involved in the misuse of spiritual teachings by the uninitiated.

A therapist, teacher, or student desiring to learn more about the teachings and practices of a specific religion can seek out a recognized spiritual teacher. Each needs to experience the results of a spiritual practice to learn how and when to use spiritually oriented techniques. This is important, as breath, mantric sound, and movement techniques can initiate profound transformative effects (Grof and Grof, 1989).

Another ethical principle is that practitioners should not force personal beliefs upon their clients. For example, if the therapist is a practicing Buddhist who attempts to influence a devout Christian with Buddhist teachings and practices, problems will ensue. The reverse of this would also apply, as would many other combinations. Respect always needs to be given to the client's preferences. Respect should likewise be given to clients lacking interest in spirituality.

DISTINCTIONS AND SIMILARITIES

The authors of the chapters in this book have bestowed ancient wisdom from the world's religious traditions. They have affirmed the deeper meaning within life and demonstrated ways to reconnect with the love, harmony, and beauty found within the heart of life. Although there are many similarities in the chapters, each has unique strengths. For example, Native traditions uniquely follow the path of the Medicine Wheel, but similar to the other wisdom traditions, they also tell stories "to let insights be passed on in a way that allows people to remember who they are." Jewish forms of meditation and holidays specifically direct us to understand the creative forces existing both within us and manifesting in the outer world. Goddess spirituality brings us back to a natural reverence for the female, unity with the earth, and respect for our bodies. Yogic mind-body practices lead to the unification or reunification of self with the universal self—to discover *So Hum* (I am that). Christianity offers a form of meditative prayer that can lead to a meaningful interior visitation by Christ, the Healer. Buddhist mindfulness meditations focus on the present moment, while the development of *maitri* (loving kindness) heals despair. Taoism specifically follows a path of detachment leading to balance. Sufism emphasizes a path to Unity through the human heart.

Many similarities are also found in the various experiential practices. For example, many wisdom traditions use stories and parables to awaken more subtle levels of understanding and awareness. They also use breath as a healing practice. In fact, a great deal of emphasis was put on breathing practices throughout this entire text. The Buddhist chapter advises the practitioner to "Let your breathing be natural. . . . If you wander away from noticing your breathing, gently return to paying attention to it." In the chapter on Christian ways of healing, Dwight Judy advises persons to take a few deep breaths to facilitate entering into a prayer state. Sheldon Kramer reminds us that breath means "spirit" and demonstrates its use in Jewish meditation. The chapter on goddess spirituality gives an example in which breath facilitated a healing process. The Taoist chapter notes that breath is a significant element of healing. In the Native American chapter we read, "As long as breath is drawn, we continue to cycle through the Medicine Wheel over and over again; hopefully, in an increasing spiral so that each time we go through the four directions, we go through them at a higher level of development and understanding." The science of breath is mentioned throughout the yoga chapter, and the chapter on Sufi healing offers a "heart awareness" meditation requiring the practitioner to breathe with an awareness of feeling.

Breath is the first and last act in life. Obviously, it is of vital importance; yet it is often ignored in psychological treatment. Breathing practices can relax stress, reduce muscular tension, and create harmony within a person, and they can open one to realization. Religious sects placing a primary influence on theology and dogma have tended to ignore the healing power of the breath and its potential to unite the practitioner with spiritual presence.

HEALING SELF, HEALING CULTURE

Throughout this century our increasing knowledge of human development has changed the way we view self, family, and community. There are many theories of psychology, and each one has contributed a great deal to understanding human development. Yet James Hillman and Michael Ventura (1992) point out in the title of their book that after 100 years of psychotherapy, the world is no better off.

Generations of familial and societal discord along with misplaced values have taken their toll. We are ready for change. We need to reconnect with the deeper meaning within life: the spiritual. It is time to take the psychological knowledge we've gleaned from the past 100 years and unite it with the thousands of years of wisdom given by the healers, prophets, saints, and mystics.

REFERENCES

Campbell, J. (1949). *The Hero with a Thousand Faces*. Princeton, NJ: Princeton University Press.

Engler, B. (1999). *Personality Theories,* Fifth Edition. New York: Houghton Mifflin.

Fadiman, J. and Frager, R. (1994). *Personality and Personal Growth,* Third Edition. New York: Harper and Row.

Grof, S. and Grof, C. (1989). *Spiritual Emergency: When Spiritual Transformation Becomes a Crisis*. Los Angeles, CA: Jeremy P. Tarcher, Inc.

Hillman, J. and Ventura, M. (1992). *We've Had 100 Years of Psychotherapy and the World Is Getting Worse*. San Francisco: HarperCollins.

Jung, C.G. (1964). *Man and His Symbols*. Garden City, NY: Doubleday and Company, Inc.

Khan, Hazrat Inayat (1979). *The Unity of Religious Ideals*. Lebanon, NY: Sufi Order Publications.

Mijares, S. (1995). Fragmented Self, Archetypal Forces and the Embodied Mind. Doctoral dissertation. UMI #9608330. Ann Arbor, MI: UMI.

Mijares, S. (1997). Narratives and Neural Winds. *Somatics: Magazine-Journal of Mind/Body Arts and Sciences,* Winter: 22-25.

Rafea, Ali, Rafea, Aliaa, and Rafea, Aisha (2000). *Beyond Diversities: Reflections on Revelations*. Egypt: Sadek Publishing.

Varela, F.J., Thompson, E. and Rosch, E. (1993). *The Embodied Mind*. Cambridge, MA: The MIT Press.

Index

Abraham(ic), 99, 101, 153
Absolute. *See also* Cosmic,
    consciousness
  a pattern, 157
  solution, 6
Abstract, 151
  reasoning, 80
  watcher, 35
Acropolis, 77
Acupuncture, 173, 174, 195, 196
Adab. See Respect
Adam, 77-78,
Addiction
  and addictive behaviors, 5, 39,154
  alcohol, 132-133, 136, 164, 219
  drugs, 133, 145
  groups for, 113
  psychotherapy for, 40, 126
  substance abuse, 164
Aggression, 86
  self-, 24-38
  and therapeutic, 32
Aging, 88-90, 91-92
Aikido, 87. *See also* Martial artists
Ain Sof, 100, 117
Air, 20
  breathing, 164
  as element, 161-162, 211, 224
  in movement, 162, 211
Ai-yai-yesh, the girl, 126-129, 137, 144
Alberuni, 208, 225
Alcohol. *See* Addiction
Allah, 156, 159, 162
Almaas, A.H., 169
Amaterasu-Omikami, 87-88
American Medical Association, 82
American Psychiatric Association, 6,
    82, 218, 225
American Psychological Association, 82
Ancestors, 82, 92
Angels, 153, 154
  Queen of, 63

Anger, 111, 116, 215, 230
  affecting liver, 178
  aggression and, 31
  assistance for, 65
  clients' experience of, 40, 60-61, 86
  healing of, 87
  hidden wisdom in, 32
Animal, 107, 182, 188
  as *nafs,* 152-154, 156
  named after, 214
  stories of, 140-142
  in twelve signs of the Chinese
    zodiac, 185-186
  wild, 154, 183
Anthropological, 72, 74
Antifeminist, 81. *See also* Misogenist
Anxiety, 86, 90, 178, 190
  Christ calming, 45, 49
  conditions that hinder, 213
  as a disorder, 229
  and fear, 3
  and the Four Noble Truths, 22-29
  to medicate, 6-8
  mindfulness of, 39-41
  outer activities, 113
Aquinas, Thomas, 81
Arabic, 89, 168
Aramaic, language of, 115
Archetypal, 101, 112, 219
  energies, 75
  experience, 3
  Goddess, 71, 84-85, 87
  initiation, 129
  maiden, mother, crone, 89-90
  psychologists, 8
  stages of growth, 230-231
Arising, 50
  in one's mind and experience, 20,
    33, 37-38
  in suffering, 21